4—

10/23

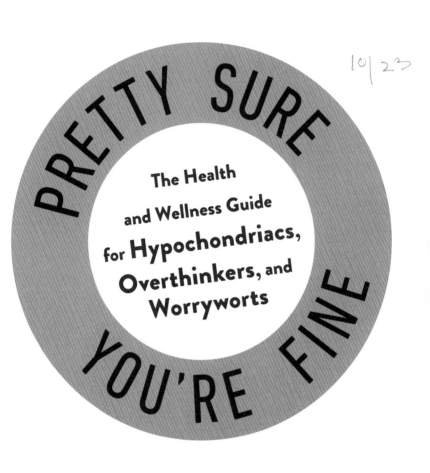

PRETTY SURE YOU'RE FINE

The Health and Wellness Guide for Hypochondriacs, Overthinkers, and Worryworts

DAVID VIENNA

CHRONICLE BOOKS

SAN FRANCISCO

Library of Congress Cataloging-in-Publication Data available.

ISBN 978-1-7972-1718-5

Manufactured in China.

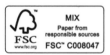

Design by Jon Glick.
Cover Design by Cat Grishaver.

10 9 8 7 6 5 4 3 2 1

Chronicle Books LLC
680 Second Street
San Francisco, CA 94107
www.chroniclebooks.com

Dedicated to my wife Larissa,
who didn't have the heart to tell me I was pudgy
until after I lost the weight.

Table of Contents

Introduction 8

Come On and Get Physical

I'm Too Tired to Exercise. 12

I Exercise, but I'm Not Losing Weight 14

Is Practicing Yoga Cultural Appropriation? 16

Gyms Are Too Expensive. 20

Fitness Boot Camp Isn't Sustainable Exercise. 22

I'll Never Look Like a Model 24

I Can't Find Anyone with Whom to Exercise. 26

Sweating Doesn't Interest Me 28

Going Totally Mental

I'm Too Distracted to Meditate. 34

I Don't Know What Mindfulness Is. 36

Is There Really Such a Thing as Stress Management? 38

Every Time I Meditate, I Fall Asleep. 40

I'm Embarrassed That I Need a Shrink 42

Can't I Just Self-Medicate? 44

I'm Too Cautious 48

Who Needs a Break When There's TV? 50

I Just Stopped By to See What Condition My Nutrition Was In

This Diet Makes Me Gain Weight. 54

Juice Cleanses Give Me Diarrhea 56

Vegetarianism Makes Me Feel Tired
and Veganism Makes Me Feel Dead. 60

I Keep Cheating on My Diet 62

I Don't Love Fast Food, It Loves Me 64

I Don't Have Time to Cook Healthy Meals. 66

I Eat Well and I Hate It 68

Do I Need to Worry about
Arsenic/Mercury/Lead in My Food?. 70

My Friend Can Eat Anything and Still Looks Great 72

Under the Lab Coat

My Home Remedy Isn't Working. 76

The Internet Says I Have a Rare Disease 78

I Need Powerful Meds to Shake This Headache. 82

My Doctor Doesn't Agree with Me. 84

I Have a Strange Pain. 86

I Haven't Seen a Doctor in Years. 88

Motivation, Inspiration, and Aggravation

Social Media Makes Me Rage 92

I Don't Know Which Wellness Routine to Start. 94

I Feel Guilty When I Nap 96

I Don't Believe in Change 98

I'm Better at Telling Others What to Do. 100

Nothing Matters, Anyway 102

Working Stiff

I Love Work More Than I Love My Kids 106

I'm Bored at Work 108

I'm Incompetent at My Job 110

My Work Stresses Me Out 112

My Boss Is Out to Get Me 114

My Employer Doesn't Care about Physical Health. 116

These Florescent Lights Are Killing Me 118

I'm Afraid It's Too Late to Report
a Work–Related Injury 120

No Laughing Matter

My Weight Affects My Health. 124

I Suffered a Debilitating Injury and Need
Physical Therapy. 126

I Have a Bad Habit That Affects Me and Others. 128

I Don't Have Health Insurance 130

I'm Depressed 132

Final Perspective 134

Sources 138

Introduction

Pretty much everyone wants to be healthy. And with a growing list of cultural and culinary movements like Pilates, hot yoga, CrossFit, mindfulness, sleep therapy, meditation, organic veggies, cage-free eggs, conscious breathing, gluten-free everything—the pressure to get wellness right can feel downright nerve-racking.

Sticking to a diet makes us eat poorly, our fitness goals are set at an unrealistic level thanks to media and advertising, and we're totally stressed out about stress. Yeah, while living a healthy life offers a ton of benefits, in many cases the pressure we put on ourselves to maintain that lifestyle ends up being counterproductive, hobbling our attempt to achieve our health goals. And when there are countless health-and-wellness gurus with 0 percent body fat shouting that we need to change, improve, break that habit, level up, try harder, longer, faster, with less food in your belly and more sweat on our brow, the pressure can manifest in destructive behaviors that are downright *un*healthy. So forget those perfectly toned windbags. They probably don't even know what it's like to spend a full half hour sobbing in the KFC parking lot while eating a four-piece combo.

Thank freaking goodness you picked up *Pretty Sure You're Fine*, because it encourages you to trust your gut (even if it's a little bigger than you think it should be), shows you things aren't as bad as you might think, illustrates how the stress you generate trying to maintain unrealistic health practices is worse than whatever your perceived problem(s) could ever be, and assures you it's okay to eat an entire sleeve of Oreos every once in a while.

This isn't just opinion. Well, it *is* opinion, but well-researched opinion by a former journalist (that's me) that is also fact-checked by a couple of totally awesome experts. Yancy Berry is a personal trainer certified through the American College of Sports Medicine and Equinox Fitness Training Institute, and an addiction recovery specialist. And Cyndi Sarnoff-Ross is a licensed psychotherapist with three decades of clinical experience, and a member of the California Association of Marriage and Family Therapists. They made sure there's no advice in here like, "Need a healthy snack? Lego bricks have zero calories!" (Even though it's true.)

Of course, *Pretty Sure You're Fine* just covers the little stuff (and some medium stuff). If your concerns involve a diagnosis of a serious medical or mental condition, please, for the love of your health, do *not* look for pointers in a book you likely found on the back of your friend's toilet.

Otherwise, feel free to dive in . . . to the book, not the toilet. For the moment, go ahead and skip the workout, break out the Doritos, and relax. Because I'm pretty sure you're fine.

COME ON AND GET PHYSICAL

I'm Too Tired to Exercise

You figure you should get in shape, but every time you think of how to accomplish this, your mind fills with a big ol' neon sign flashing one single word in glowing red letters: *exercise*. Just saying the word wears you out. Like, why so many syllables, ex-er-cise? Why can't it be short and fun, like *eat* and *sleep*?

And you dread making time during the day to run or swim or—even worse—ride a Peloton bike. You have stuff to do, after all. There's work, and those back episodes of *Law & Order: SVU* aren't going to watch themselves.

No amount of caffeine can break through the wall of exhaustion and procrastination you're stuck behind. You wake up tired every morning, sleepwalk through the day, and collapse on the couch each night. You're so tired, even your naps leave you needing a nap. The herculean effort required to create and maintain an exercise routine that would benefit you in any substantive way would take more energy than you have to offer.

Pretty Sure You're Fine . . .

We all push ourselves too much a lot of the time. We work through lunch, let vacation days go unused, and end the day just as exhausted as we started it. Being tired all the time is pretty common (one study found that 40 percent of all Americans wake up tired multiple times a week). In that way, there's nothing wrong with you—or rather there's nothing unique about that particular affliction.

But here's something you might not want to hear: Exercising regularly can help you sleep better and increase your daily energy. Yeah, just hearing that makes you want to have a little lie-down.

Leave the CrossFit madness to professional wrestlers and Marvel movie actors.

Don't worry about becoming a triathlete overnight. Start small with a daily walk and give yourself time (months, not days) to see and feel results. As the walk becomes easier, add distance or increase your pace. And leave the CrossFit madness to professional wrestlers and Marvel movie actors.

I Exercise, but I'm Not Losing Weight

You glance in the full-length mirror (something you normally avoid) and notice you're a little thicker around the middle than you realized, and you'd like to fit into your favorite pair of pants again. Or maybe it wasn't even your idea. Maybe your doctor advised you to lose weight, the jerk.

But after weeks of exercise, you still look like an overstuffed Hostess Twinkie. So, you adjust your schedule to make it more of a priority. Weeks later, you still look doughy and gross. What the heck? It's common knowledge exercise makes you into an Adonis. But, no, not you.

Nope. It's best to just buy new, slightly larger pants and settle into your current form, one that's sort of doughy and always creaks when you stand up.

Pretty Sure You're Fine . . .

As our bodies age, our metabolism slows. It's just nature taking a well-deserved cool-down after sprinting groin-first through puberty. It's unrealistic in your forties to maintain the same chiseled physique you may have had during your twenties. So, some extra pounds are usually okay.

If your doctor advised you to lose weight, however, you should probably listen because they went to school for this and you went to school for, what, anthropology or something? The fantastic news is *exercise* means a lot of different things and most of them aren't painful. You don't need to go from lazing on the couch to flipping a tractor tire in the gym parking lot overnight . . . or at all, really.

You don't need to go from lazing on the couch to flipping a tractor tire in the gym parking lot overnight . . . or at all, really.

It's possible that you're not seeing results because it's just too soon. Sometimes it takes months to see real effects of regular exercise. Of course, there are other possible reasons: Real, lasting weight loss comes when you couple exercise with dietary changes; everyone's body is different and yours just might like to take things slow; you're exercising too much (yes, that's a thing); you're not being 100 percent honest about your calorie intake; and/or you're not doing the right *kind* of exercise (an alternating combo of cardio and strength training tends to work best). And body fat percentage is often a more important metric for tracking progress than actual weight loss. Some people who do weight lifting or calisthenics can see a reduction in body fat with no change (or even an increase) in weight. If you're interested in tracking your progress accurately, try a scale that also approximates your body fat percentage.

In the meantime, don't sweat the weight (see what I did there?), and just keep lacing up.

Is Practicing Yoga Cultural Appropriation?

You think yoga might be for you because it looks like a lot of posing and staying still, which seems far less stressful than all of that running/cycling/weight lifting claptrap. Y'know, the kind of exercise seen in Gatorade-sponsored posts with muscled athletes screaming as they sweat through their workout. Yoga seems like the opposite of that: lots of quiet contemplation and very little sweat. But you're not sure if yoga is a religious thing, or a cultural thing, and if it is, is it inappropriate to participate?

Pretty Sure You're Fine . . .

Yoga's roots are pretty firmly planted in the Hindu religion. The Sun Salutation is how Hindus traditionally greet the Sun God Surya, for example, and when you turn to your yoga buddies and say "Namaste," you are literally saying, "The god in me bows to the god in you," which is an acknowledgement of a divine power. So, unless you worship *that* god, a case could be made that you're not just participating in cultural appropriation, you're participating in religious appropriation as well, which might not be worse, but it feels like it probably is. Y'know, like if you went around baptizing random people just because you felt the spritz of water might cool them off on a hot day.

Of course, no one's going to know if you and your pals create an underground yoga class, like a fight club for the Whole Foods set. And there are some who believe focusing solely on the physical aspects of yoga might not be that bad, the same way atheists still celebrate Christmas, but at that point you might as well add a pose called Splitting the Hair because that's what you're doing. (Oh, and the same goes for tai chi, which has its roots in religions like Confucianism and Taoism.)

You might as well add a pose called Splitting the Hair because that's what you're doing.

I'm pretty sure you're fine, however, because there are plenty of low-impact exercises that offer similar benefits as yoga, such as Pilates, Callanetics, or swimming. And the only way to offend anyone while swimming is if you poot in the pool.

A Bit of a Stretch: Yoga Alternatives

Most modern yoga techniques combine physical stretches, breathing exercises, and mindfulness meditation to create a whole mind-and-body wellness practice that also occasionally makes you fart unexpectedly. But, since you're a sensitive, well-meaning person, you were swayed by the warning that practicing yoga very likely *is* cultural and religious appropriation (page 14). So, here's a deep dive into the aforementioned yoga alternatives and a few others that are sure to leave your whole mind-and-body wellness practice offense-free.

Pilates: Created by Joseph Pilates as a physical rehabilitation technique for soldiers returning from war, this type of workout focuses on small movements to both strengthen and relax core muscles. Many of the exercises include (or can include) breathing techniques and meditation, practically making it yoga's secular cousin who sometimes doesn't get invited to family gatherings.

Callanetics: Developed by former ballerina Callan Pinckney, this technique (which draws on both ballet and yoga, minus the religious aspect) focuses on small muscle groups which are worked in "bursts," repeated movements with limited range of motion. It's meant to tone and strengthen certain muscles, and if you're looking for cardio, seekest thou elsewhere, because this technique is so low-impact, it's basically no-impact.

Swimming: Not sure this needs to be explained, but just in case, swimming is when you get in the water and make like a fish. Widely considered a great full-body workout, the environment and fluidity of movement tends to minimize injuries and is therefore especially helpful for those recovering from injuries or with other physical conditions. Also, it's the rare combo of low-impact *and* cardio exercise.

Dance: Whether contemporary, ballet, or some combination of various forms, such as barre, dance offers a unique and—let's admit it—fun way to work certain muscle groups. Throw in a little meditative contemplation of the music and you've got yourself a yoga alternative you can dance to. (Slam dancing is not recommended.)

Stretches: No longer just for the moment when you first wake up and yawn, stretching routines offer benefits similar to yoga—working core muscles, increased range of motion, and helping prevent injuries. You also don't need to join a studio or burn incense to do it.

Parkour: This one's probably better for those looking for an alternative to extreme yoga because parkour involves jumping, diving, leaping, flipping, crawling, and hurling yourself up, over, and under various obstacles. Think of it like an elementary school playground speed-run.

On a final note, one aspect of yoga that makes it so popular is that combination of physical exercise and meditation. But, really, you can really add meditation to any exercise . . . except maybe the javelin throw.

Gyms Are Too Expensive

One of those big fancy gyms opened up in your neighborhood and you think maybe getting yourself to a place specifically to exercise might help you actually get in shape. Gyms have all that fancy equipment too, so you could even break up your workout like the fitness pros do. You could have a "leg day," whatever that is.

You tour the place and are not disappointed. The treadmills, weights, and ellipticals gleam almost as bright as the staff's hairless triceps. Then, the toned salesperson shows you a rate sheet and your heart rate ramps up to a speed faster than any workout could possibly produce.

With these prices, you'll lose weight simply by selling off less-vital organs to pay for the membership.

Pretty Sure You're Fine ...

Way back in the Paleolithic Era, there was a guy on TV named Jack LaLanne. He was a huge hit with all the cave dwellers. His whole thing was that you can exercise literally anywhere. (Technically, that would include free-falling from an airplane because, yes, you can do abdominal crunches while plummeting at 200 feet per second.) He would demonstrate how to use things like a chair or a doorway to do simple routines to stay fit. And if you think he was some crusty old Boomer, firstly, he was part of the Greatest Generation, so he was older than a Boomer and, secondly, that guy worked out every day until he suffered muscle failure. Every. Day.

All that is to say, you really don't need a gym to work out. Calisthenics, like push-ups and sit-ups; strength training exercises, such as yoga or weight-lifting; and countless other forms of exercise don't require any special equipment. Nor do they require pounding EDM blasting from the room's sound system.

With the money you save by skipping a gym membership fee you can buy yourself something nice, like a private jet.

Need weights? Use a couple of laundry detergent containers. Don't have a yoga mat? Try the floor. Can't afford a treadmill? There's a whole world outside in which you can run, and the scenery is probably way better than the walls of your unfinished basement. With the money you save by skipping a gym membership fee, you can buy yourself something nice, like a private jet.

Fitness Boot Camp Isn't Sustainable Exercise

You want to kick-start your exercise routine, and what better way to do that than with a fitness boot camp. Heck, boot camps work for the military, and a bunch of glistening celebrities swear by them to lose weight and tone up fast as well.

So, you sign up and get started. And the fitness instructor yells at everyone over their little PA system to push harder, run faster—it's fantastic and exactly what you need. That is until the second day, when your muscles uncontrollably shake, followed by the third day, when you blow out both of your knees, which makes even the simple act of standing upright a painful endeavor.

Your body is clearly way more of a lost cause than you thought. If a few days of intense workouts can do this much damage, there's no hope for you to ever get fit.

Pretty Sure You're Fine . . .

While the intensity of fitness boot camps may be what you're looking for, what you'll statistically find instead is a collection of injuries. That's because people who subject themselves to high-intensity workouts like this without any prior fitness training are more likely to hurt themselves, even in actual military boot camps, where nearly 30 percent of recruits suffer a training-related injury. That's right, boot camps even hurt our brave soldiers.

The little irony these flashy boot camp advocates sometimes forget to impart to potential clients is this: Boot-camp-style workouts work better for those already in shape and who are looking to increase their fitness regimen. The Mayo Clinic warns, "Boot camp exercises usually involve ballistic, rapid movements that can be too challenging to those who aren't already in shape."

It's not that your body *won't* handle a boot camp workout. It's that, if you're kick-starting an exercise regimen, your body needs to work up to it. Just like there's no pill to help you safely lose weight, there's no skipping the steps for creating an exercise routine for yourself. So, start smaller.

If you're kick-starting an exercise regimen, your body needs to work up to it.

Take your time. The boot camp will be there when you're ready. And when you *are* ready, still take it slow—one or two classes a week with days to rest between. (Besides, muscles tone when they're recovering from workouts, not during them.) As you progress, you can increase the number of workouts until you're a boot camp pro or drill sergeant, or whatever they're called.

I'll Never Look Like a Model

You do everything right. You diet, you exercise, you stay up on the latest fitness trends, you meditate, and you're so freaking mindful that when you do a crossword puzzle you can literally hear your brain's synapses firing like a string of black-market firecrackers. And yet, when you look in the mirror, you look nothing like Gigi Hadid or Bella Poarch. What. The. Heck.

Your waist size won't come down, your arms remain flabby, and your thighs are staging an active revolt against logic and decency. If only your body would do its part, you, too, could be a TikTok megastar or an Instagram influencer. But no, your body refuses to play along. The best you can hope for it is to become mildly popular on a forgotten platform like LiveJournal.

Pretty Sure You're Fine . . .

You undoubtedly know this, but it bears repeating: Models, celebrities, and influencers set an unrealistic standard and employ a whole brigade of makeup artists, stylists, groomers, publicists, photographers, and trainers to make themselves look flawless, and a host of media headlines to make you forget all of that. Yeah, it takes lots of work to look like you don't do lots of work.

And there's biology and physiology to consider. Even if you mimic someone's diet and fitness routine exactly, you'll still likely get different results because, to put it quite plainly, you are not them. (Though, experts don't want you to use that as an excuse to avoid your health.) Also, consider the time spent working on your body. You may head to the gym after work, but for many of these celebrities exercising in the gym *is* their work. In fact, Justin Gelband, a personal trainer for a number of former Victoria's Secret models, says, "You can't compare somebody who has been working out their entire life to somebody who hasn't."

It takes lots of work to look like you don't do lots of work.

If you're healthy, that's fantastic and you should be proud of yourself. If you're working on it, keep at it, but don't make a superstar your goal. Make yourself your goal.

Shut Your Pie-Hole

You may want to strike up a conversation at the gym and, if you find a similarly chatty person, there's nothing wrong with a little mid-workout banter. But, here's a shortlist of phrases and questions you should never ever utter:

- My parole officer suggested I do this to work out my anger issues.
- Do you want to bench me?
- I need to power through this workout because my newborn is in the car.
- I heard they built this gym on an ancient tribal burial ground.
- Where is the smoking section?

I Can't Find Anyone with Whom to Exercise

Let's face it, you are a social person. You like to hang with friends, you dig the camaraderie you feel with your coworkers at the office, and you believe a good cocktail goes better with a drinking buddy. So naturally, getting in shape would be much more fun if you had a partner, someone to cheer you on as you do for them. But when it comes to finding that person, you get no takers. It's all crickets and tumbleweeds. And the crickets are already in shape.

You don't want to be alone in this quest, quietly wiping away tears as you do squats or penning morose poetry in your head as you cycle through your Pilates routine. It's best to just avoid solo workouts altogether. Maybe you could just do some burpees at the bar while your drinking buddy gets the next round.

Pretty Sure You're Fine . . .

There's something to be said for doing some wellness practices alone. Like, sure, group meditation exists, but why? That said, exercising with other people has benefits, such as increased motivation, consistency, and experimentation.

You don't need to let your lack of takers affect your health. If you want to exercise with people, there are tons of classes—such as yoga, spinning, CrossFit, Jazzercise . . .

Sure, group meditation exists, but why?

Wait, is Jazzercise still a thing?—that offer you the group dynamic you crave. And, according to a 2010 study in the *Journal of Social Sciences*, working out with a group could increase the effectiveness of whatever exercise you're doing because your fellow classmates' habits may positively influence you.

If you're not into classes, you could try jogging in the local park (if there's one nearby), even though it might not be the exact same thing as having a friend jogging alongside of you. Many parks have public exercise equipment and trails, which are often full of similarly active people, as well as at least one drifter shouting angrily at a trashcan.

Who knows? You might make a few new friends, y'know, ones that won't bail on you just because you mention breaking a sweat.

Bring It Home

There are plenty of ways to get in shape at home without selling a kidney or a child to afford equipment. Look around your home. Trot up and down the stairs outside of your apartment a few times for your very own StairMaster®. Lift cans of soup like weights for a few reps. And get more bang from your pushups by employing a basketball to balance on. Just don't ask your teacup chihuahua to spot you.

Sweating Doesn't Interest Me

Sweating is gross. You know it's natural, but lots of natural things are gross. Ever seen mold? Or a banana slug? Sweat makes your hair clumpy, your skin clammy, and your clothes stinky. Really. Super. Gross.

Plus, doing the work that makes you sweat is hard and ridiculous. Running? No thanks. CrossFit? Yeah, right. If getting in shape means you must sweat, you can just tell exercise to stick that stationary bicycle up its callipygous caboose.

Where Truth Lies

There are so many myths about physical fitness, they might as well put a gym in Area 51. Here are two biggies:

- "Muscle weighs more than fat."—Untrue. A pound of iron weighs the same as a pound of feathers. A pound is a pound is a pound. Muscle, however, is denser than fat. That's why you may actually not lose weight (or even gain weight) when losing fat.

- "Shred every day to build muscle."—Nope. Your muscles don't form and grow when you work out. They do that when you stop. So, if your goal is to tone up, give your muscles a day or two to rest during the week or at least rotate which muscle groups you work each day.

Pretty Sure You're Fine...

There are those who say the more you sweat, the more calories you burn. These people are what's known in the scientific community as "wrong." In fact, one study showed that you burn the same number of calories in a 90-minute Bikram yoga class as you do on a brisk 90-minute walk.

When you imagine adding exercise to your routine, it's natural to think of extreme workouts and Nike ads with athletes covered in rivers of perspiration. But it's important to keep in mind that literally any physical activity burns calories. That's what calories are for. So, depending on duration, things like walking, Pilates, or tai chi simple stretches can cut your calories and even help tone your body as effectively as other forms of exercise without leaving you all sweaty and stinky.

And there are plenty of actual workouts and sports that are nearly or completely sweatless, such as ice skating, swimming, and aerial yoga. Even if you want to push yourself a little more, you can employ some simple tricks to get a better workout, like speeding up parts of your workout (sounds counterintuitive, but it's true) or resting between sets. Sadly, power napping doesn't burn as many calories as its name suggests.

Weights and Burpees and Squats, Oh My: The Best Exercises Ever

You've decided to start exercising regularly instead of just counting your semi-daily sprint for the city bus. But, from work to errands to critical vegging-out periods, your time is precious. (Experts suggest thirty minutes of exercise a day, five days a week.) So, you want to be sure that you make the most of it with the best possible workout. Well, *huzzah!* And for added emphasis, *abracadabra!* Here are some of the most recommended exercises by fitness professionals.

Weights: Don't worry. *Weights* doesn't mean you need to clean and jerk a barbell loaded with 400-pound discs. No, modest dumbbells will do fine. (And if you are in the market, look for the adjustable kind, so you can add weight over time.) Reps of simple curls or overhead presses will help build and tone muscle. Dumbbells can also be added to lots of different exercises—like lunges and walking—to increase the workout benefits. Do not, however, try to multitask by bringing dumbbells into the shower. Trust me, I know from experience.

Burpees: Despite the cute name, this exercise will kick your butt. And your legs. And your stomach . . . It will kick your everything. That's because burpees literally work every muscle in your body. There are plenty of videos online to show you exactly how to do them, but here's the basic cycle: squat, plank, pushup, back to plank, jump up, jumping jack, repeat. After thirty to sixty seconds of that, you'll start to think of less cute names for it, like Pain Maker or Just Kill Me Now.

Squats: Ah yes, the tried-and-true squat. They key to getting the most out of these (without damaging your back) is to keep your shoulders back and engage your core muscles. Squats work everything below your chest and, like burpees, require no equipment or even clothes. Yeah, you can do squats in the buff, if you want. Just close the shades first, okay?

Yeah, you can do squats in the buff, if you want. Just close the shades first, okay?

Increasingly popular high-intensity interval training (HIIT) workouts include various strength-training exercises such as these. Weights, burpees, and squats are all considered "strength training," rather than "cardio" activities such as running or swimming. Cardio helps decrease fat, strength training helps build muscle, and both burn calories. So, for general fitness that includes weight loss, experts suggest a workout that combines the two styles. And, of course, food intake affects the success of any exercise regimen. So, the benefits of that fifteen-minute HIIT session gets obliterated if you celebrate with a cinnamon roll, or four.

GOING TOTALLY MENTAL

I'm Too Distracted to Meditate

The benefits of meditation seem like something you could get behind—reduced stress, more focus, better mood. And it's free! No food program to buy into, no gym to join. Just you, the couch, and some serious breathing.

Yet, whenever you sit to get your meditation on, your mind goes into overdrive. Your brain fills with a cacophony of thoughts, images, and questions: If cowboys are adults, they should be called cowmen. How do we know there are colors we can't see? Loraine really can't pull off those penny loafers, and she should know that. How much does a blanket cost? Celery smells like body odor. Can a monkey learn to drive a car?

The effort of clearing your mind simply made room for all the stupid thoughts your typically busy mind kept at bay. And you suddenly realize how twisted your brain actually is. You'll never get to experience the benefits of meditation, at least not until after you learn whether or not a monkey can drive a car.

Pretty Sure You're Fine . . .

Meditation isn't just about clearing your mind, though that's a huge part of it. It's a skill, and like any other skill you need to practice to get better at it. For some, mastering meditation can take months or even years. Experts suggest you not fight the distractions, but welcome them, examine why they're popping up, then move on. This is the mindful part of learning to meditate. Accepting that distractions will happen (with less and less frequency as you hone the skill) makes the process less frustrating.

And if you still find it an insurmountable task, you're not alone. In fact, some people find being alone with their thoughts so insufferable, they'd rather receive an electric shock.

Happiness Is for the Dogs (and Cats and Birds and Fish)

Your furry friend offers more than companionship and the occasional slobbery lick. Science says having a pet improves your overall health. And why would science lie? Petting your animal pal lowers your blood pressure, walking them can help you lose weight, and a study found that 74 percent of pet owners reported "improved mental health." That's worth an extra treat.

I Don't Know What Mindfulness Is

You've heard the buzzword, you've seen it on T-shirts, mugs, and hand-painted signs meant to hang in your kitchen. But *mindful* means about as much to you as *nude trampoline calculus*.

Maybe it means thinking about every step of your day, but you tried that and for a few harrowing seconds you forgot how to breathe. Maybe it means thinking really hard about stuff, which you already do about a lot of stuff, especially that one time the grocery clerk said, "Thanks for shopping with us," and you replied, "You, too!"

Your brain is already spinning with work deadlines, shopping lists, your kids' practice schedules . . . adding mindfulness to that hodgepodge of stress sounds hard and exhausting. In fact, you could probably stand to try a little mind*less*ness.

Pretty Sure You're Fine . . .

People throw around the word *mindfulness* with the same frequency and accuracy as words like *cool, literally,* and *Sir, pants are required to enter the store*. So, just to get it straight, to be mindful means to be aware of your present state, which includes what you're doing and how you're feeling, with acceptance and without judgment.

According to psychotherapist Cyndi Sarnoff-Ross, it can even increase your sense of pleasure. She suggests a simple and tasty exercise to help draw your attention inward: Put a piece of chocolate in your mouth. Instead of just swallowing it, close your eyes, notice not just the taste, but also the texture, how it dissolves, the sound your mouth makes, the smell. See there? You've just mindfully eaten chocolate.

Let's say a task at work makes you mad. Mindfulness allows you to acknowledge and even explore the negative feelings while experiencing them and how they relate to the task. Think of it as an occasional "Why you mad, bro?" asked to your heart by your brain.

For most of us, being totally Zen in the moment, every moment, is about as realistic as using a bowling ball to play table tennis.

And it's a skill (a type of meditation, really) you must develop, so don't get down on yourself if you can't get the hang of it. For most of us, being totally Zen in the moment, every moment, is about as realistic as using a bowling ball to play table tennis. So, don't pressure yourself. There are alternatives to mindfulness such as breathing-based mediation. Those can put you on the same path to improvement without the pressure of acing mindfulness out of the gate.

Is There Really Such a Thing as Stress Management?

Work, bills, your health, that late-night text from your ex, the weird noise your car started making, the fact that everyone you follow on Instagram seems to be having a much better time and more colorful cocktails than you—all of it stresses you the heck out. You've got to get this under control.

But how? You've tried puzzles, baking, karaoke, bingeing Korean game shows, wine, naps, and even a visit to a spa and none of it alleviates the hiking backpack of stress you feel every day. On top of that, it's affecting your sleep, which, irony of ironies, adds stress.

Relax With a Hobby

Do you need a therapist if you have a hobby? I don't know, I'm not a therapist. Jeez. But, studies show that hobbies and activities such as drawing, dance, cooking, and gardening are fantastic for your mental health. Research also revealed that hobbies are "linked to lower levels of depression and may even prevent depression for some."

You pour yourself another large helping of chardonnay and hope that one day the stress will just go away. Because managing it can't be done.

Pretty Sure You're Fine . . .

Stress, even a large amount of it, is actually pretty common. So, don't let the fact that you're stressed stress you out. A trip to a spa or just shutting off your brain with some mindless TV can help. But, if those aren't doing the trick, there are some other things you can and should employ.

Don't let the fact that you're stressed stress you out.

According to the Mayo Clinic, exercise, meditation, even laughing reduce stress and anxiety. So, hit a comedy club every once in a while. Maybe jog there if you can. Of course, there's no shame in seeking professional guidance from a therapist, either. There are many different types of therapy to choose from, such as cognitive behavioral therapy and group therapy, so you can find the one that suits you best.

Oh, and when it comes to stress, a glass of wine or a cocktail is okay, but multiple glasses increase stress, both on your body and your ability to sleep soundly. So, keep that in mind . . . unless you're meditating, in which case clear it from your mind.

Every Time I Meditate, I Fall Asleep

You shut off the laptop and kick off your shoes. It's time for your daily meditation, something you're proud to have added to your routine. Because that means you care about your health and mental well-being. In fact, you'd pat yourself on the back right now, if it weren't time to get meditating.

You close your eyes, breathe, and feel the calm flowing from your lungs to your stomach and neck, then to your arms and legs. Your mind is clear, and your body is relaxed. You're such an absolute master of mindfulness, you think you may have surpassed historic meditation guru Maharishi and gone all the way to full-fledged Jedi.

You realize you weren't in the midst of a meditation so much as a power nap.

When your head bonks against your desk, however, you realize you weren't in the midst of a meditation so much as a power nap. The bruise forming on your forehead joins the others from previous days. And you realize you actually suck at this meditation thing.

Pretty Sure You're Fine...

It's okay to be sleepy or even doze off. If the goal of meditation is inner peace and you're at peace when you sleep, hey, mission accomplished. If you'd like to be conscious for your meditation, however, there are a few simple things you can do, like moving to a new spot (definitely stay away from meditating on a bed) or meditating with your eyes open. Try focusing on posture—spine erect, shoulders back, chin slightly down—that can also help you keep the *zzzs* at bay.

And look, meditation isn't for everyone, and it isn't easy. Sometimes, the struggle to get the hang of it can actually *add* stress. Perhaps you need to find another activity instead, whether it's simple physical exercise, doing a puzzle to exercise your brain, or trying to get through *Finnegan's Wake*.

Also, you might want to examine your sleep schedule. Are you getting enough and is it restful? According to the Mayo Clinic, you should be getting at least seven hours a night. If you've had a few cocktails before bed, for example, the full night's sleep you get won't be as restful as the same amount of time minus the multiple nightcaps. Plus, waking up rested feels as good as being drunk, anyway.

I'm Embarrassed that I Need a Shrink

Your neighbor started exercising regularly and not only lost twenty pounds, but also says she handles stress better than ever. Your coworker started meditating and says it's the best thing she's ever done for her mental well-being. You'd be happy for them if it didn't already have your brain spinning with anger and jealousy over their improvements, adding stress you didn't need to your already stressed life.

Everybody's so into self-diagnosis and self-care, they're like a chatty Facebook wellness group. You don't know exactly what's wrong with you, though, and you feel like you need some expert help. But, seeing a therapist signals to everyone that your brain is just broken. How could you show your face at the office Christmas party if they're all going to be whispering about your need for a shrink?

Maybe, to fix all of this, you need to quit your job and become a mountain hermit whose only friends are squirrels and gophers that would never judge you for anything except your berry consumption.

Pretty Sure You're Fine . . .

First of all, your brain is not broken. Brains literally can't break. If anything, they'd smush. But no actual breaking would happen. So, let's just nip that little untruth right in its annoying bud. And while some forms of self-care can do wonders, sometimes you really do need something besides a turn on the elliptical machine and ten minutes of meditative silence.

Repeat this phrase to yourself: Seeking professional help *is* self-care. Good, now say it again.

Repeat this phrase to yourself: Seeking professional help *is* self-care. Good, now say it again. And again. Repeat it until you believe it because it's true, it's important, and it can help.

Plus, as psychotherapist Cyndi Sarnoff-Ross points out, the idea that seeing a professional therapist means you're crazy is as antiquated as thinking leeches will cure a cold. (Note: They won't.) Not only is therapy wildly common, you also don't have to have a diagnosable mental health disorder to take advantage of it. In fact, doing so actually demonstrates power and dedication to yourself.

It's not only a popular form of mental care, but it also offers more than just a person to whom you can get things off your chest. It can help in ways you probably haven't even considered, such as giving you an advocate, a new perspective, and tools to (here it is) do some real self-care. And even better, it can help prevent stress from becoming a more serious mental health issue.

So, put away your unwarranted embarrassment. You can totally see a shrink without shame. (Just don't call them a shrink. That's a big no-no.)

Can't I Just Self-Medicate?

Sure, you're stressed out, tired, and deal with occasional bouts of anxiety, depression, and general malaise. You're a typical human person after all, not a superhero. But all the self-help techniques people spout on about are simply ridiculous. Cycling doesn't raise your spirits; it just makes you tired and sweaty. Therapy doesn't alleviate your stress; it alleviates your wallet of cash.

Anyway, you've got a much better way to take care of yourself. A bit of weed, maybe a cocktail, perhaps a Zoloft aperitif. What's the harm in a little muscle-loosener now and again or a few puffs of green? (Aside from the late-night fridge raid, that is.)

All that stuff is *mostly* legal, or, depending where you live, *completely* legal, and it works to push your stress away for a while. So, pop a pill and spark a joint. You've got it covered.

Pretty Sure You're Fine . . .

Yes, the benefits of marijuana, specifically cannabidiol (aka CBD), has become quite a popular way to prevent "the long-term adverse effects of stress" and treat various forms of anxiety. Though the professionals who advocate for medicinal marijuana do *not* suggest turning your apartment into a gigantic Kush hotbox. (Also, marijuana use has been associated with the exacerbation of depressive symptoms, which means using weed to "treat" these things might actually be making it worse. Just sayin'.)

The professionals who advocate for medicinal marijuana do *not* suggest turning your apartment into a gigantic Kush hotbox.

And if you've got Zoloft or some other beta blocker, hopefully you got it using a prescription that came from a licensed doctor and not some guy named Dingo Dan who hangs out behind the Arco station on Route 32. Beta blockers, which slow the heart rate and block the effects of adrenaline, not only reduce stress but also can "blunt the negative effects of stress and anger on people with a history of atrial fibrillation."

So, while some components in weed can be helpful, and a medical professional might think you'd benefit from a prescription medication, the same can't be said of alcohol. A drink now and again is okay, but drinking away your stress or anxiety is never a good solution for all of the reasons you surely already know from watching your brother-in-law get blasted during Thanksgiving dinner and telling your mom what he really thinks of her.

When it comes to why you might be self-medicating, the best question to ask yourself is: Are you self-medicating to numb feelings? If so—especially if you can't stop or feel regret afterward—you should strongly consider addressing those underlying issues. Especially if you invented a cocktail and named it My Therapist.

Who Thunk It First?: The Origins of Mindfulness

Mindful meditation, mindful work, mindful yoga, mindful relationships, mindful cooking—your mind is full of mindfulness. It started as a buzzword and now it's a complete movement that claims to help you improve your mental, emotional, and even physical health. We're not going to go into what exactly mindfulness means (for that, see "I Don't Know What Mindfulness Is" on page 34). Instead, let's look at its roots, which date back nearly 2,500 years, which means it is, in fact, older than Jesus.

Like yoga, the origins of mindfulness can be traced back to ancient Hinduism, though the folks who created it back then weren't aware of the future need for succinct marketing catchphrases, so rather than call it mindfulness, they called it Dhyāna (meaning "contemplation"), which hopefully leads to samadhi ("a state of meditative consciousness"). Of course, Hindus didn't have a total lock on the practice. Almost at the same time, Buddhists began doing their own version with the goal of reaching nirvana, which, contrary to what you might think, was not solely a kick-ass grunge rock group from the '90s, but also a mental and spiritual state of pure knowledge akin to listening to a kick-ass grunge rock group from the '90s.

While there are a few instances of Eastern practitioners bringing mindfulness to America in the early 1900s, and even some Western religions incorporating their own version of mindfulness throughout the intervening couple of thousand years, it really didn't hit the United States in any familiar way until the 1970s.

That's when University of Massachusetts professor Dr. Jon Kabat-Zinn created a program called Mindfulness-Based Stress Reduction (MBSR), which he based on the Buddhist meditation practice called Vipassana. MBSR focused on the mental and physical health benefits, making mindfulness a tool for doctors. And it hit at the exact right time because in the '70s everyone was looking for the next big self-improvement craze and most of them had pretty much learned that disco and cocaine didn't work.

Now, there are just as many applications for mindfulness as there are types of sandwich condiments.

Now, there are just as many applications for mindfulness as there are types of sandwich condiments. And picking the version that works for you depends on whether you're more of a Dijon mustard person or a ranch dressing person, mindfully speaking.

I'm Too Cautious

You feel pretty healthy. You take care of yourself, eat right, and exercise. There was that one time you rode your bike down to the coffee shop without a helmet, but that was a rare occurrence in an otherwise danger-free life.

Your best friend, however, celebrated her first BASE jump by downing the better part of a bottle of Jose Cuervo and tried to teach herself parkour by leaping from her second-floor balcony to the parking garage without any safety gear whatsoever. And your manager said he tried blowfish at the local sushi joint the other night just for the thrill of it. Blowfish! That stuff can kill you if you get a chef with a shaky hand.

What is with these reckless daredevils? Don't they understand life is fleeting and death is fickle. Or maybe, you just need to lighten up a bit. Yeah. Maybe you should cut loose a little. You could drive to work without a seatbelt or eat that leftover tuna salad that's been sitting at the back of the fridge for two weeks. Look out, people. There's a new risk-taker on the scene. Now, hand over that blowfish, pal.

Pretty Sure You're Fine . . .

This has been said a lot, but it bears repeating: Never, ever, under any circumstances, compare yourself to others. Just as everyone's body, metabolism, health, and even odor is different, so is everyone's comfort level.

Never, ever, under any circumstances, compare yourself to others.

Don't be jealous of your BASE-jumping friend, especially if you've never had the desire to hurl yourself from a high-rise into the great abyss. You, as they say, do you.

If you do feel envious of the more cavalier people in your life, look for ways to broaden your experiences gradually and in a manner you feel comfortable. Just BASE jumping (to run further with that example) right away would be too much of a leap (pun most definitely intended), so maybe head to the nearest amusement park and ride that coaster that you always wanted to try.

And there are benefits to leaving your comfort zone, besides increasing your heart rate and need to pee. According to psychiatrist Abigail Brenner, MD, challenging yourself can help you tap unused knowledge and personal resources, as well as make you better at handling change.

Who Needs a Break When There's TV?

Everyone tells you that you should exercise or meditate, if for no other reason than to clear your head at the end of the day. And, sure, that might work for them, but you have other, more entertaining ways to clear your head. Namely, Netflix, HBO Max, Hulu, Amazon Prime, and a whole host of other services that give you access to pretty much everything that's ever been shot, edited, and streamed.

Sweating through abdominal crunches sounds way worse than binging that new crime drama about that small-town detective who's trying to solve a murder. You know that one in which everyone talks in a funny Pennsylvania accent. Ooooh! Or the show that takes place in Elizabethan England, but the cast is really diverse and they just have a bunch of sex.

Yeah, you wouldn't have time to exercise or meditate even if you wanted to. Popcorn?

Pretty Sure You're Fine ...

When it comes to the benefits of meditation, there's at least one study that claims "mindfulness" is about as effective as just watching TV. The thing to note, however, is that what types of shows you watch can play a part in how well they help you relax and clear your head.

You see, when you watch a show, your brain is still working, just not like it usually does. Typically, your neocortex (where reasoning and analysis happen) shuts down, but the visual cortex, the brain's largest cortical tissue, is highly stimulated. So your brain's working, it's just that nothing comes of it, kind of like that novel you keep not writing.

So your brain's working, it's just that nothing comes of it, kind of like that novel you keep not writing.

Other studies show that intellectually stimulating shows, like documentaries or fact-based series, relieve the guilt of watching TV, whereas "guilty pleasure" shows (ones we know are bad, but we love them anyway) often leave us feeling, well, guilty. And that increases stress, rather than alleviating it. Like with those casual self-medicating substances, if you're zoning out to avoid or numb feelings, you should probably address that. The Elizabethan sex show can wait.

I JUST STOPPED BY TO SEE WHAT CONDITION MY NUTRITION WAS IN

This Diet Makes Me Gain Weight

You've tried every diet trend—Paleo, grapefruit, South Beach, Atkins, cabbage soup—and not one of them has had the desired effect of immediately making you look like a waifish twenty-two-year-old Instagram influencer. And now that you've found one and decided to really stick with it, it's not only not having the desired effect, it's having the *opposite* effect. You're gaining weight.

What in the actual hell, diet? While celebrities touted this as the way to shed pounds, your pants get tighter with each passing day. And on top of that, you're constantly hungry. And not for a snack. No, you could see yourself tackling an unsuspecting fast-food mascot and devouring that clown in a few horrific bites like some sort of pudgy zombie.

You're clearly a failure at this whole magic diet thing. You might as well resign yourself to the fact that your body will never change. You're destined to live out the remainder of your sad days at this weight . . . unless, of course, you gain more.

Pretty Sure You're Fine ...

Not every diet works for everybody and some of them, if not monitored by a nutritionist, can lead to a "diet cycle" (which sounds fun, but is actually nothing like riding a bike) or worse, serious health issues such as heart disease or infertility. So, take whatever diet advice you got from whichever reality star with a grain of salt. Yes, even if you're trying to cut out salt.

Take whatever diet advice you got from whichever reality star with a grain of salt. Yes, even if you're trying to cut out salt.

The good news is you're not helpless. There is a myriad of reasons why you might be adding instead of dropping weight. If you're coupling your diet with exercise, you may be gaining muscle. Other common dieting mistakes people make: Incorrectly tracking calories; continuing to drink sugary drinks; not "counting" alcohol, which is generally very high in calories.

If you've accounted for all these possibilities, you might want to check with your doctor to determine if a medical condition might be hindering your weight loss and how to address it. Otherwise, keep at it and stop drooling over that clown.

Juice Cleanses Give Me Diarrhea

Cleanses are good, right? When you clean your apartment, your poker buddies say things like, "The place looks great!" and "Did you hire a maid or something?" You just sit back and beam with pride over the cleanse you performed that garnered all this praise.

You decided to apply a similar technique to your body to give your new health regimen a kick start. And a juice cleanse sounds like the way to go because, hey, you like juice. You bought the books, read the articles, got the ingredients, and broke out the blender you haven't used since your Cinco de Mayo party.

After downing a couple of concoctions, however, your body seems to want to put this cleanse into overdrive by evacuating everything south of your lungs as quickly as possible. You now have an entire library resting on the side of your tub since you now spend huge blocks of time on the toilet, and you need something to occupy yourself. At least you're catching up on that book club list.

Pretty Sure You're Fine . . .

When it comes to juice cleanses and detoxes, there are a lot of factors to consider. One such factor: Diarrhea tends to be a perfectly common side effect of them. Nutritionist Ilyse Schapiro warns, "You may find yourself running to the bathroom much more often when you're on a juice cleanse, even though you're consuming so much less than usual." (And it should be noted that the other side effects, such as bad breath, lethargy, and possible ongoing digestion issues aren't fantastic either.) But, if you're just worried that your keister keeps singing "Ol' Man River," the culprit is likely a lack of fiber. So, y'know, have a side of broccoli with that kale smoothie.

Also, not every diet or detox technique functions the same on everyone. Consider the possibility that you should try other forms of cleanses or whether you really need one at all. You might see better results faster by skipping the pre-regimen detox and going straight to your regimen.

Lots of Appeal

Bananas make you happy and not just because people can slip on the peels, which—let's face it—is just a classic gag. The squishy yellow fruit is packed with vitamin B^6, which the body uses to make serotonin. And that's important because serotonin positively affects your emotional stability, motor skills, sleep—all of which help combat depression.

Vegetarianism Makes Me Feel Tired and Veganism Makes Me Feel Dead

Whether for health or environmental reasons, or just because you love all creatures great and small, you decide to make a pretty drastic change to your diet. You want to aim for a vegan lifestyle, but you think starting out with a simple vegetarian one might ease the transition. Goodbye, rib eye steaks. Hello, tater tots.

But after a week or so of potatoes and cheese pizzas, you feel lethargic and fuzzy-headed all of the time. Your strength has gone the way of your beloved bacon swiss burger. You decide to forge ahead and cut out dairy, honey, and anything else that can be traced back to a living creature. You did it. You are now a full-tilt vegan. And you're miserable.

Maybe we were meant to eat living things. Because the alternative feels like a slow, bland death.

Pretty Sure You're Fine . . .

Unless you were raised vegetarian or vegan, switching up without doing any research or creating a nutrition plan can lead to failure and even health issues. In that way, it's very much like performing an organ transplant. So start by consulting with a nutritionist.

You'll find, if your metabolism is accustomed to high-protein meats, you can't just ditch them like you did that clog-dancing-enthusiast you met on Bumble. You need to *replace* them. Find good sources of protein, like nuts or beans (many of which provide different kinds of protein that you can mix to form complex proteins). Or try having a plant-based protein shake once or twice a day in addition to protein-rich foods.

If your metabolism is accustomed to high-protein meats, you can't just ditch them like you did that clog-dancing enthusiast you met on Bumble.

Also, you don't have to go from zero to Moby in one go. A pescatarian diet—one in which you cut out meat and poultry but keep fish and shellfish—is a healthy way to stagger your nutritional journey. And whether you choose to aim for a pescatarian, vegetarian, or vegan diet, the benefits are countless and include lower blood pressure, lower cholesterol, and less inflammation, all of which mean improved heart health, a reduced risk of developing diabetes, and a reduced risk of certain types of cancer.

I Keep Cheating on My Diet

The otherworldly euphoria you feel sneaking a Hostess Twinkie between meals fades away as you realize the damaging effect it has on your nutritional goals. Most days you can maintain the right schedule, foods, and calorie count. But sometimes, the siren call of Ben & Jerry's Salted Caramel Brownie ice cream drives you straight to the freezer with a spoon and a craven expression. And all it leaves you with is a cold chill of failure and a restart date for your diet.

Why is dieting so freaking hard? Why can't you tell your body, "Listen, private. We're cutting back on carbs and sugar," and have your body salute and reply, "Yes, sir! I will shoot carbs and sugar on sight!" To which you'd probably reply to your body that shooting a gun at carbs and sugar might be a bit extreme and where the heck did that rifle come from anyway?

Whatever. It doesn't matter. You weep quietly as you finish the cinnamon roll and lie, yet again, to your calorie tracking app.

Pretty Sure You're Fine . . .
Diets are hard, man. Like, for real. Especially those cravings. Those things are *powerful*. That's because

you're literally jonesing for a sugar or fat high. Dietitian Beth Czerwony explains, "Our brains are chasing that pleasurable state of food euphoria."

Everyone struggles when they change their eating habits. They are habits, after all. But, in addition, your body becomes accustomed to certain things—saturated fats, sugars, etc.—and simply jettisoning them from your meals can lead to frequent falls (and, sometimes, spread-eagle leaps) from the diet wagon.

That doesn't mean it's impossible. You just need to employ some tricks, some biological slight-of-hand, if you will. Experts suggest you never let yourself get hungry during the day—always have a healthy snack at the ready to avoid feeling the need to pig out. Another suggestion is to get sleep and to meditate because stress makes it harder to avoid those cravings. And a no-brainer piece of advice: Don't keep junk food in the house. Like, you wouldn't send a Labrador to live in a beef jerky factory, no matter what a good boy he is.

You wouldn't send a Labrador to live in a beef jerky factory, no matter what a good boy he is.

I Don't Love Fast Food, It Loves Me

You know you should cut back on the fast food, but, man, a Big Mac would sure hit the spot right now. And what's the harm, anyway? One measly combo meal a few times a week can't be that bad. If it was, it'd be regulated, right? Like, they have warnings on the sides of cigarette packs and alcohol ads warning us to "drink responsibly." Surely, sweet ol' Wendy would wag her little finger at you for ordering a Bourbon Bacon Cheeseburger Triple if it were *really* unhealthy.

As you peel open that Taco Bell Grande Crunchwrap, you decide to be safe and walk around the office once or twice, to burn a few more calories. That'll do the trick.

Pretty Sure You're Fine...

Here's the deal: One or two fast-food meals a month is okay-ish. People generally stress about their daily calorie intake, but some suggest looking at it by week instead. Sure, you had a greasy burger for lunch Tuesday, but the rest of the week you ate healthy. Your body can handle that, like a Cheat Day meal. In fact, giving yourself a predesignated cheat meal every couple of weeks helps you psychologically as well because it gives you something to look forward to. So, if that's what you're doing, yes, I'm pretty sure you're fine.

If not, though, you need a different book than the one you're reading now. Because there is no "healthy" fast food. All of it is dangerously high in sodium, fat, and sugar. And to burn off the 1,280 calories in the aforementioned Wendy's Bourbon Bacon Cheeseburger Triple, you'd need to do more than walk a couple of extra times around the office. You'd need to walk about 10 miles. And if you're having meals like that multiple times a week, you are at risk of heart disease, heart failure, obesity—you know, fast food's greatest hits.

Not only that, but a 2018 study found that "eating processed foods and fast foods may kill more people prematurely than cigarette smoking." So, uh, congrats, fast food. You're now worse than cigarettes.

A homemade burger is typically lower in calories and fat than one made by a clown.

Consider packing your lunch or making meals at home, which dramatically decreases the negative stuff. Unsurprisingly, because you're in charge of the ingredients, a homemade burger is typically lower in calories and fat than one made by a clown or a jack-in-the-box.

I Don't Have Time to Cook Healthy Meals

Between your work schedule, the kids' activities, your housework, and making sure the dog gets out for a walk so he doesn't leave a revenge poop in the dining room again, you have no time—not a single minute—to cook an actual meal. Sure, you can microwave the heck out of some soup or a pizza. But when it comes to fancy home-cooked meals, you can only get those at a restaurant, preferably one that delivers.

That's why they invented fast food—for people like you who need food, uh, fast. Let those professionals stand at the griddle and work the deep fryer, you've got crap to do. Maybe, if you work hard and long enough, you can hire a chef to make meals for your family. You do the math and determine you may be able to achieve that in . . . 93 years. Better grab a handful of potato chips and get to it.

Pretty Sure You're Fine . . .

First of all, you are not alone. Sociologists found that modern unpredictable work schedules and other factors make finding time to cook increasingly difficult for pretty much everyone. (We could get into how every-thing seems to suck all the time and, for that reason, whether or not it's even worth it to be healthy, but that's for later in the book. Go ahead and crank that emo playlist to get yourself ready, though.)

Go ahead and crank that emo playlist to get yourself ready, though.

But, if you *can* squeeze in just ten minutes, you could make a healthy home-cooked meal. There are literally tens of thousands of one-pan or slow-cooker recipes that take mere minutes to prepare. (Think hearty dishes like chili or shrimp pasta, or lighter fare such as lemon chicken or sausage quinoa.) And, if you get your family involved in the prep, it speeds things up even more and becomes a fun activity for all.

And if that's still too much time for you, prepared meal delivery services offer healthy options without all the chopping and mixing. They're not cheap, but neither is eating out every night nor paying for whatever cholesterol meds you'll need later.

A Funny Thing Happened on the Way to Healthiness

Laughter makes you healthier. Whether you snicker, chuckle, or guffaw, the act of laughing lowers your blood pressure, helps prevent heart disease (by improving vascular function), and even helps fight off illness. So, go ahead and let loose at whatever awful joke your partner made. It'll literally make you feel better.

I Eat Well and I Hate it

You eat lots of salad, drink plenty of sugar-free liquids, and skip dessert. Your nutritional intake sets the bar for health. You account for every calorie, every gram of fat, every grain of salt. And you hate it. Not just hate, you loathe it. It *suuuuuuuuuuuuuucks*.

You want to take the food you eat and nutrition guides you've read and toss them into a woodchipper perched on the edge of a fiery volcano. You long to have a thick steak and a heaping side of greasy french fries followed by a towering sundae smothered in chocolate syrup. You fantasize about dancing in a shower of donuts and fettuccini Alfredo. You yearn to run up to anyone who ever claimed to like brussels sprouts, grab them by the lapels, and scream into their face, "Who hurt you?!"

Yeah, eating healthy sucks. At least you can eat junk food in your dreams.

Pretty Sure You're Fine . . .

You eat healthy? Wow, good for you. That's an impressive feat.

If you're not enjoying it, however, you probably just need to give yourself a break. Cycling through the same smattering of meals over and over can get monotonous, especially if they all taste like off-road tires. So try lightening up on your own restrictions. Sugar, saturated fats, salt—small amounts of these won't make you suddenly unhealthy. Bored with the avocado toast or rice cakes? It's okay to have a strip of bacon or a hamburger every once in a while.

It's okay to have a strip of bacon or a hamburger every once in a while.

You might also try an international flair. Some of the many notoriously healthy and flavorful cuisines from around the world include Mediterranean, Japanese, and Indian food. That's because these diets tend to lean more heavily on vegetables and seafood, rather than American fare that typically features meat and has higher amounts of fat and sodium. And, seriously, if they could run for office, Americans would elect fat and sodium president and vice president.

Ultimately, just try to remember why you made this commitment. Doing something as simple as focusing on the goal rather than the process can affect your palate and mental state for the better.

Do I Need to Worry about Arsenic/Mercury/ Lead in My Food?

Your mom sent you an article that claimed high levels of arsenic are found in rice. You bookmark that in the folder where you have other articles she sent you about aliens running the government and Elvis living in Belize disguised as a cabaret performer.

But something about it bugs you, not because you think it's another load of your mom's ridiculous paranoia, but because you know it could be true. You already know about mercury in fish and lead in water. After those revelations, you gave up sushi and tap water. Now, you're taking omega-3 supplements and you've gained a couple of cavities.

Cutting out foods seems to have just as bad of an effect as ingesting the bad stuff. Still, one more such discovery and you may have to give up eating just to stay alive, if you call that living.

Pretty Sure You're Fine . . .

Let's tackle these one-by-one, shall we? First, fish. Specifically, mercury in said fish. Yes, some fish contain high levels of mercury. But, to paraphrase clueless bros

This Is Nuts

You probably never knew that decorative container of walnuts your parents set out anytime you had company was like a bowl of bitty brown brain boosters. That's because walnuts make you smarter. While nuts are already high in healthy fats and protein, walnuts specifically have a lot of alpha-linolenic acid (that's good for your arteries), and one study found eating walnuts in particular increased cognitive function.

---

on Twitter, "not all fish." Salmon, cod, tilapia, catfish, and a bunch more are way low in mercury (or have none at all). And other seafoods like shrimp, oyster, and crab are okay, too. And to get a real case of mercury poisoning, you'd have to eat fish high in mercury, like, every day for a couple of weeks. And only sharks do that and that's why sharks are high in mercury.

Now, lead in tap water. Believe it or not, unless you have lead pipes in your home, this shouldn't really be a concern. However, if you do have lead pipes or if you're concerned because that's just the kind of worried person you are, most inexpensive carbon-based filters remove pretty much all lead from tap water. So, drink away.

Finally, the arsenic thing. Yes, arsenic occurs naturally in the soil and a small amount of it does get into rice. With this, Andy Meharg, a professor at Queen's University Belfast and arsenic superfan, feels it's all about how much rice you eat. He says, "It's dose-dependent— the more you eat, the higher your risk is." So, don't freak out about it, but don't go on a rice binge either.

My Friend Can Eat Anything and Still Looks Great

You're watching your weight, trying to make good food choices. At a kid's birthday party where the only options are veggies with ranch dip or greasy pizza, you choose raw broccoli sans dip. The mom of the birthday boy, though, wolfs down three pieces of pepperoni with extra cheese and chases it with a Mtn Dew. Worse, she eats like that all the time. Even worse, she looks like a JLo backup dancer.

While you're forced to graze at vegetable trays like a vegan bovine, she's out there delighting in plates of spaghetti carbonara like she's carbo-loading for a 10K. And should you ever risk the rare nibble of a patty melt or french toast, you inflate like a Macy's Thanksgiving Day Parade balloon. It seems even *smelling* a slice of red velvet cake makes you gain back the three pounds you lost last month.

You exercise until your lungs burn, you measure your food intake ounce by demeaning ounce, you drink more water than a trout. It feels like an extraordinary effort with little gain for all the trouble. You wipe a drop of drool from your chin as you watch your friend dip the pizza crust in the ranch and enjoy her delicious carbs.

Pretty Sure You're Fine . . .

You understand everyone's body is different, right? Well, the same goes for everyone's metabolism. And the way in which everyone wears their weight. Some people have to work harder to stay fit, while others don't seem to have to work at all, the cretins.

Despite what you've undoubtedly heard, metabolism plays less of a part in weight gain or loss than calorie intake. Not only that, but the director of the Nutrition & Metabolic Health Initiative at Texas Tech University, says, "by nature of having more mass, a larger person burns more calories," which means a heavier person has a higher metabolic rate than a thinner person. (That's why, when you do lose weight, it seems harder to lose more.) And according to the U.S. Institute of Medicine Subcommittee on Military Weight Management, you have absolutely zero say in most of the things that determine your body weight, anyway, "including developmental determinants, genetic makeup, gender, and age." So, focusing on metabolism alone is like worrying about the quality of gin served on the Hindenburg. . . . Sorry, probably not a good time for a blimp reference.

Focusing on metabolism alone is like worrying about the quality of gin served on the Hindenburg.

Here's something else to consider: You don't know exactly what other people's lives are like or what they do with their time. Let's take your friend enjoying the pizza at her kid's birthday party. Sure, she may have the body of a seventeen-year-old water polo enthusiast, but she may also go home or to the gym after the party and work out for three straight hours.

So the absolute worst thing you can do is compare your metabolism or body type to that of anyone else. It's like comparing an elm tree to a Buick Skylark. Rather than seethe with jealousy over how other people maintain their health with supposed ease, it's best to focus on what works best for you. Discuss a plan or technique with your doctor, a physical trainer, or a dietician. And keep in mind that you likely won't land on the right strategy right away. But, if you keep at it, you'll find the steps that work for you, and then someone else can seethe with jealousy over you.

That Burning Sensation: Making Calories Work

Regular exercise can sometimes seem monotonous. It is "regular," after all. If you're looking to throw in some irregular exercise, however, you're in luck. Because pretty much every activity burns calories, even knitting. Seriously, just fifty minutes of working on that holiday scarf for your neighbor uses 100 calories.

Feeling lazy? Great! Certain forms of laziness actually use a substantial number of calories. A 160-pound person sitting in front of the TV for an hour will burn 81 calories and their post-show nap burns 45. And if you don't know what to do with your hands, fidgeting can blow through up to 350 calories in a single day.

Of course, you're undoubtedly wondering about the ol' horizontal mambo, so let's start at the beginning. Blinking burns 2 calories per blink. So flutter those eyes, lover boy, and watch the pounds disappear. If those come-hither looks end up attracting a suitor, maybe offer a massage. Giving someone a shoulder rub for forty-two minutes and you'll burn through 200 calories. If that leads to sexy time, you'll end up burning way more, 101 on average for men and 69 for women. (Yes, I see it, too. It's just a number. Let's move along.)

And though it's not recommended, enjoying a postcoital cigarette burns 10 calories. Of course, if you experience any burning elsewhere after sex, you should seek out a salve or something. Unfortunately, there's no reliable data on exactly how many calories you'll use applying it.

UNDER THE
LAB COAT

My Home Remedy Isn't Working

Your mom always knew the best cure for a cold was chicken soup and plenty of daytime TV. So when the seasonal bug going around the office finally caught up to you, you loaded up on Campbell's offerings and fluffed the pillows. Yet, despite downing at least three bowls over the course of two days, you're not feeling any better. Maybe you should've made your own soup like Mom used to because this canned stuff isn't doing the trick.

On top of that, while heating up your latest helping, you burned your finger. When you applied your mom's standard home remedy of butter, nothing changed. Your finger still hurts like heck. In hindsight you realize that butter never did anything for your burns except make them smell delicious. It's time to accept the fact that your mother is a fraud and a liar.

Pretty Sure You're Fine . . .

Your mom's not evil, just a little misinformed. Many home remedies are derived from myths and lore that do not stand up to scientific scrutiny. Putting butter on a burn, for example, has no beneficial effect and, because treating a burn includes letting the area cool, smothering the injury with a substance like butter may make recovery take longer.

That said, some home remedies do actually work. Treating nausea with ginger or muscle pain with mint, for example, are scientifically proven. And according to recent studies, even treating a cold with a bowl or two of chicken soup has some anti-inflammatory benefits and aids in the movement of nasal fluids.

Your mom's not evil, just a little misinformed.

So, sure, battling a cold means you are, by definition, probably *not* fine. But if your home remedy isn't working, it might just mean that you need to switch to a remedy based more on science or that your cold is simply—and this is a technical term—a "doozy" that chicken soup alone can't ward off.

Futurists Promised Us a Pill That Cures Everything

That magic pill we were promised is probably rotting away in the glovebox of the flying cars also promised to us. But, fear not! The leaps and bounds of modern science and medicine means conditions incurable just a few years ago now have an expiration date. There are a ton of existing and improving cures for whatever ails you, with recent advances in medications for HIV, Alzheimer's disease, hepatitis C, cystic fibrosis, and others. Even the Big Casino—cancer—is currently looking down the barrel of a solution. So, no, there's not one magic pill. But, a few pills and a couple of injections ain't bad.

The Internet Says I Have a Rare Disease

You woke up feeling a bit off and after searching your symptoms on various medical websites, message boards, Reddit, and one BuzzFeed quiz entitled "Which 16th Century Disease Are You?," you're now convinced you have either ameloblastoma, neuroacanthocytosis, or Jumping Frenchmen of Maine. (And, yes, that latter one is the real name of a real disease.)

You're no alarmist, but it's all there in black and white and sometimes accompanied by an animated GIF. The internet said so. And why would the internet lie? Sure, it missed the mark entirely with that whole Y2K bug and, no, Slender Man is not real, but whatever. These deceptively mundane symptoms mean you are destined to leave a legacy as a biological mystery, as a chapter in a medical textbook, a freak of nature, a dire warning of the power of DNA's wrath.

Women will gasp as you pass by, shuffling slowly through the streets of foggy old London (never mind how you got here, just go with it). You'll crane your misshapen form to the night sky and cry, "I am not an animal! I am a human being!" Of course, that one website said crying into the night sky is likely a symptom of something called fingelhausertosis. So, you're totally screwed.

Pretty Sure You're Fine...

Unless you went to medical school, you're no doctor. And the only types of doctors that don't need multiple years of training, a license, and certification are '70s rock musicians, certain brands of soda pop, and comic book supervillains. Before he turned to evil, Doctor Doom wasn't, like, a podiatrist or anything.

Speaking of evil, a study published in *JAMA* found that medical communication companies (aka websites like *Web*MD and its ilk) "receive substantial support from drug and device companies." Yes, the dreaded Big Pharma. I'm not saying they stand to make more money by making you think you're sick, but I'm not, *not* saying it.

Also, the accuracy of diagnosis on those sites varies wildly and is never 100 percent accurate. So the bruise on your arm may be just a result of bumping it in the night, but a site called something like CarnivalofFatalDiseases.com may suggest you have an alien parasite. And you've seen enough movies to know there's no cure for that particular ailment that doesn't end in a spontaneous involuntary C-section.

While seeing your symptoms listed on a page, describing what happens to you when you have cancer or diabetes or even something super rare, like Wandering Spleen (again, real thing), you should keep in mind that things such as sore throat, aches, stiffness, and congestion are extremely common. Sure, a headache could mean cancer, but it could also mean you just need to drink more water. If you're concerned, the best course of action is to seek the opinion of a medical professional. Just make sure it's not Doctor Doom.

A site called something like CarnivalofFatalDiseases.com may suggest you have an alien parasite.

Psychology Potpourri: Intro to Lesser-Known Forms of Therapy

You've heard of hypnotherapy and maybe thought that was a little out there. But, man, you ain't heard nothing yet. While the numerous benefits of therapy are nothing to scoff at, some of these unusual types of mental analysis and healing are so weird, it may leave you . . . well, needing therapy.

Your mental health is no game, unless you want it to be. If so, you might want to seek out **Chess Therapy**. This technique employs the age-old game to build a relationship between patient and therapist as well as help clear the mind.

If you want to keep it light after checkmate, give **Puppet Therapy** a whirl. Created by occupational therapist and Jim Henson–wannabe Ingrid Lagerqvist, this technique uses puppets to get children (and some adults) to open up about trauma and other issues.

Sand Therapy is the only form of mental health that gets into all your cracks and crevices. Invented by Dora Maria Kalff, a Jungian psychologist, this form of therapy encourages patients to literally play with sand to induce calm, which assists in clearing the mind and creates a literal physical connection to their surroundings.

If communing with nature's your thing, consider **Wilderness Therapy** (you and your therapist go for a hike), **Horticulture Therapy** (you and your therapist garden together), or **Equine Therapy** (taking care of a horsey *is* your therapy). But, if you really want to let it all out, you should try **Nude Psychotherapy**. Psychologist Paul Bindrim took an idea by nudist Howard Warren and just ran with it. Naked. The idea behind (hee-hee, I said *behind*) this practice is to strip down our defenses and let it all hang out.

And look, these all may seem weird to some, but not everyone likes sand or puppets. Whatever form of mental health practice works for you, please do it with no shame, no fear, and, in the case of the last technique, no clothes.

I Need Powerful Meds to Shake This Headache

Your headache won't seem to go away. You tried ibuprofen, naproxen sodium, aspirin, and even a head rub from your massage-hobbyist roommate, but nothing will knock this dull pressure away. That's when your buddy has an idea: Just try one of her pain relievers. She promises it's the high-octane stuff, prescription-only and sure to do the trick.

Despite a childhood spent watching various after-school specials and a few "very special" episodes of normally hilarious sitcoms, you consider it. It's not like you're a drug addict. Not yet anyway. Is that how this all starts? "The first one's free," the pusher always says. Oh, my God, is your friend a drug dealer?

Pretty Sure You're Fine . . .

Okay, Hold a beat. Do *not* take whatever horse pill your friend gave you. Especially, if your friend is an actual horse. The doses those creatures take could drop a . . . well . . . a horse. Throw the pill in the trash. Now, if your headache has gone on for an afternoon or a day or even a couple of days, there are perfectly logical and simple reasons why you can't shake it, none of which should lead to taking strange drugs.

If you're under a sizable amount of stress at work or at home, for example, that may manifest as a lingering headache. If you aren't sleeping well or drinking alcohol right before bed (you don't have to go to bed drunk to experience the joy of a hangover), that could be the cause. Not drinking enough water, eating too much sugar or sodium, or even a change in the weather can spark a headache. None of those triggers is a reason to do your own version of *Fear and Loathing in Las Vegas*.

Instead, try to sleuth out the root cause and address it. Nurse practitioner Shannah Young suggests "keeping a headache diary to track characteristics of your headaches," which will help your doctor narrow down possible causes and fixes. Other fixes include exercise or meditation for stress; better sleep practices; eating better and staying hydrated; treating potential allergies. Neurologist Dr. Ronald Andiman says, "If your headaches are increasing in frequency or severity, or are interfering with your usual activities, see a doctor." The same goes if the headache goes on longer than a couple of days or you experience vomiting. Otherwise, you're likely okay.

My Doctor Doesn't Agree with Me

When you felt a little tightness in your chest, you did the responsible thing and saw your doctor right away. Well, not before a little internet research and a klatch with some trusted friends. You were sure you could save the doctor's time by explaining that you know you need an MRI, a CT scan, some bloodwork, and whatever other tests they have because you're sure you have heart disease. Or a brain tumor. One of the two. Or both.

But, after checking you over and asking a few questions, your doctor forgoes all the fancy machinery and tests and prescribes some exercise and a vacation. It seems your doctor thinks the tightness in your chest is just run-of-the-mill work stress. Well, what the hell does that quack know? Time for a second opinion or multiple opinions, whatever it takes until you find someone who comes to the same, very obvious conclusion as you.

Pretty Sure You're Fine . . .

You're expecting this section to tell you that you're right to seek another opinion. Nothing's stopping you. Go. Have fun. It's your money. But that's not why I'm pretty sure you're fine.

I'm pretty sure you're fine because the licensed doctor who went to years and years of medical school and literally knows more about this than you said you're okay. Even if one or all your friends went to medical school, they're not *your* doctor, who knows your medical history, your stresses, your diet, your blood type, and where you got that weird fungus last summer. The truth is misdiagnoses are pretty rare. A study of diagnostic errors in outpatient care found they happen at a rate of just 5 percent, and only half of those are even harmful.

That said, the key to a useful doctor-patient relationship is open communication. If you don't feel informed when visiting with your health care provider, don't hesitate to ask for more information or clarification. If your doctor recommends something you legitimately don't want to do—like a medication with severe side effects or a referral to a specialist outside your insurance network—don't be afraid to bring up your concerns. Cardiologist Dr. Steven Nissen says, "Be straight up. Look someone in the eye and say, 'I've greatly appreciated your care over the years, but this is a big decision and I'm not sure about it. Is there someone you can recommend who can see me to give me an independent opinion?'"

Of course, you can be *too* overcommunicative. Don't, for example, tell your doctor about your expansive WWE action figure collection, especially during a colonoscopy.

I Have a
Strange Pain

It just appeared one morning. You woke up, stretched, and one of your back muscles (or maybe a muscle cluster?) got angry at you and staged an immediate revolt in the form of a shooting pain so acute, you thought for a second your cat had fashioned a shiv and stabbed you for buying the cheap kibble.

Once the initial pain settled into general soreness, you felt confident in getting out of bed. That was your second mistake (just after waking up in the first place). The dull throb hung around like your former college roommate who crashed on your couch during that two-day EDM festival then stayed an extra week "just to catch up."

A tweaked muscle is one thing, but this lingering ache inevitably means something big, maybe catastrophic. You'll try over-the-counter pain relievers, then switch to the hard stuff, then end up getting arrested for trying to knock over a pawn shop for cash. You should've just stayed in bed.

Pretty Sure You're Fine . . .

Let's face it, you're no spring chicken. You're barely a fall chicken. At best, you're a midwinter chicken. And even if you are in your prime, sometimes weird aches or pains just happen. It's your body's way of showing you who's boss. Think it's your brain? Oh, no, pal. Think again. And see if all that thinking can avoid a thigh cramp.

Muscle aches, pains, even sprains can sometimes just happen, the cause of which is often either stress, vitamin D deficiency, dehydration, or poor sleep. Of course, there's also overuse or underuse of said muscles. That's why statistically most back injuries occur when good Samaritans agree to help their neighbor move their new recliner upstairs. (That statistic is not true at all, but you get the gist.)

Most back injuries occur when good Samaritans agree to help their neighbor move their new recliner upstairs.

If you can press on the muscles and reproduce the pain, you likely have a physical injury or sprain, and back pain, specifically, can also be your body's SOS for a few different things, so don't ignore that. But, if those are ruled out, you need to *really* worry about those strange pains only if they're accompanied by dizziness, shortness of breath, fever, nausea, vomiting, or urinary changes. Or, if your cat has been giving you dirty looks for not getting Fancy Feast.

I Haven't Seen a Doctor in Years

You went through a financial rough patch a few years ago and had to tighten your purse strings a bit. That meant cutting out nonessentials like dining out, upgrading your phone, getting an extra credit card, and buying mid-shelf or higher pinot noir. Things eventually righted themselves, but until you caught a nasty cold, you totally forgot you'd also stopped going to your regular physical. In hindsight, it's a miracle you didn't need any emergency care that whole time, especially considering how you pushed the envelope with those sell-by dates on the food in your fridge.

You imagine returning for a much overdue checkup and discovering your doctor doesn't even know you anymore. Sure, there's a glimmer of faint recognition in his eyes, but it soon passes as he scans your tests. Then, those eyes fill with concern. If only you'd come in a year or just a few months earlier, something could have been done. But, no, your negligence toward your health made your body a veritable carnival for a host of diseases and viruses, all of which should finish ravaging your system within days, maybe hours.

Pretty Sure You're Fine . . .

You are not alone. A 2021 study by OnlineDoctor.com found that nearly 20 percent of Americans have not had a doctor visit in five years or more. That's one out of every five people! That means at least one person in your book club is *way* overdue for a checkup.

Of course, that study also found that 23 percent don't trust their primary care physician, which is a whole other problem. If you're one of those people . . . y'know, switch doctors, for goodness' sake.

The amazing thing about your body is when something's wrong it'll usually tell you. If you've had chronic conditions or a sudden change in your health, get thee to a doctor. But even if not, it's probably time to strap on the gown and get checked from soup to, uh, nuts. And you can optimize your appointment by doing things like asking for a longer appointment and prioritizing your list of concerns. And don't forget to schedule a dental cleaning, too, because, let's face it, your breath smells like a yeti's armpit.

> It's probably time to strap on the gown and get checked from soup to, uh, nuts.

MOTIVATION, INSPIRATION, AND AGGRAVATION

Social Media Makes Me Rage

Your aunt posted a picture of a sunset over a lake on Facebook, and it popped up on your feed. It would have been lovely if not for the glaring text on the photo, which read, "Go out on a limb. That's where the fruit is." Squinting at the image, your brow furrows. It contains no limbs, no fruit. Just a lake, probably full of fish poop.

You stand and start to pace the room as you try to deduce whether she meant that for herself or for everyone else. If it was for her, why post it on social media? Why not just read it, take the sentiment in, and move on? No, she probably thinks this is some grand wisdom and posting it in her senior quilters' Facebook group makes her look like Buddha or John Mayer.

As you pulse starts to quicken, you remember your coworker's Instagram post that showed her lounging by a pool at some Mexican resort, cocktail in hand, #Blessed. Meanwhile, you were cleaning up dog vomit from the living room rug because your terrier accidentally ate one of your Steve Madden sandals and it didn't agree with him.

What was clearly intended to inspire or uplift you now has you in a full-tilt rage spiral. If you needed empty platitudes and saccharine experiences, you'd have cracked open a fortune cookie. At least those taste good.

Pretty Sure You're Fine...

You don't need this book to remind you that too much time spent on social media is bad for you in more ways than you think. If you do, though: Too much time spent on social media is bad for you in more ways than you think. Overdosing on Facebook, Instagram, TikTok, Twitter, and the like can lead to depression and jealousy, and even keep you from achieving your own goals.

Of course, not everyone gets sad when confronted with what appears to be constant evidence of people who are living their best life and telling you how to do it. Some get mad. And some want to toss their laptop into a ceremonial bonfire. Psychotherapist Dr. Aaron Balick says, "In some cases [social media] may be an accelerator, increasing the anger, frustration, and polarization that is already there."

Like with anything that pisses you off, be aware of your triggers.

So, if social media is pissing you off, that's okay. Just make sure you don't let that rage go unfettered. Like with anything that pisses you off, be aware of your triggers. If your aunt or coworker's posts regularly upset you, simply mute, block, or unfollow them (and keep the snarky subtweets to yourself).

I Don't Know Which Wellness Routine to Start

Okay, you're prepared, you're motivated, you are freaking *pumped*. Today's the day you make a change for the better. Today's the day you kick off a new healthier you. Your water bottle is full and you're ready for action . . . but, what action?

Should you focus on a mindful routine? Meditation always sounds good. Wait. Isn't yoga also a kind of meditation? Or you can meditate while you do it? Or is that mindfulness? Ugh. You haven't even started and you're already stressed out.

Maybe you should concentrate on physical health. Yeah, body first, then you'll worry about mind. So, some cardio seems like a good way to start. Running, no . . . swimming, yeah, swimming would be great. Except there isn't a pool nearby. And quite honestly, if you have to drive to a pool, you likely won't keep up with the routine. There's that CrossFit gym that just opened up. . . . Wait, is CrossFit cardio or strength training? Or both. You think it's both. Is that too much wellness?

Dang it! Forget it. You collapse onto the couch, tired and sweating from just trying to figure out how pick the perfect routine for you. You figure you were meant to shirk any wellness process and just keep ignoring your mind and body. Ignorance is bliss, after all. Maybe it can be health, too.

Pretty Sure You're Fine...

When you consider the sheer volume of possible health and wellness regimens that are available, it's easy to feel overwhelmed. That's normal, especially if you haven't already landed on some sort of routine. So, here's why you're probably fine: You don't need to land on the perfect routine right away. It's your health, not a driver's test.

Start with what you want to do. Want to roller skate? Strap on those wheels and go, kid. Once you're out there moving and having fun, you'll find it easier to experiment with other forms of exercise or add less desirable workouts. Or just keep it super basic. For physical health, simple stretches and light cardio help get things started without leaving you sore from an afternoon grunting at the gym. The same goes for mental health. Meditation is a skill you must hone, not an activity you just do. It takes time to get the hang of it, so take it easy on yourself if you get distracted, especially if you have a cat, because when they want a scratch behind the ear they don't care if you're struggling to be mindful.

When it comes to improving your health, look at it as a journey rather than a destination.

Also, when it comes to improving your health, look at it as a journey rather than a destination. Executive coach Jody Michael writes, "It's less about reaching your goal and more about recognizing progress along the way." But you knew that because you're smart and you've read some Ralph Waldo Emerson.

I Feel Guilty
When I Nap

Does the body really know what it needs? Right now, it's saying, "Shut the laptop, sneak out to the car, and pass out in the back seat for thirty minutes." But maybe that's just the bread and cheese you ate for lunch talking, inducing a food coma. Maybe your body needs to fight the sultry pull of the nap and do something to wake up, like a walk around the block. How do you know when to listen to your body and when to go the other way?

I mean, your stomach tells you when you're hungry and it's never wrong. Your dry mouth tells you when you're thirsty. Your armpits tell you when to shower. And right now, your brain—not just your brain, but your very core—is calling for rest and a little shut-eye. Babies do it all the damn time and you are definitely pro-baby.

Pretty Sure You're Fine . . .
Look, napping is perfectly fine and healthy. A little recharge often helps improve things like focus, mood, even digestion. Never fear a nap.

However, if you did just eat a large meal and you did have a good night's sleep, then the signal your body is sending you is probably mixed. It's saying, sure, napping is an option, but so is walking around the bock twelve times to pump fresh blood to that sleepy brain of yours, especially if you haven't moved your bones yet today.

Of Fame and Fitness

Lots of actors dipped their perfectly manicured toes in the world of fitness. Before he traveled back in time to hunt Sarah Connor, Arnold Schwarzenegger made his name as the youngest Mr. Olympia champion. And right around the time when she was working *9 to 5*, actor Jane Fonda so enjoyed her personal fitness routine that she created a series of instructional home videos and a cultural movement. And before Billy Blanks created the Tae Bo workout, he kicked his way through some low-budget martial arts flicks.

Dr. Michael Grandner, director of the Sleep and Health Research Program at the University of Arizona in Tucson, says a power nap "can improve memory and reduce fatigue for the rest of the day." However, if you need a lie-down because you can't stay awake, it could mean you're not getting enough decent sleep at night. If that's the case, behavioral sleep medicine specialist Dr. Shelby Harris suggests you see a doctor to confirm there aren't any medical issues keeping a good night's sleep at bay.

There's also an epic irony in the fact that people who exercise have more energy. So, if you feel lethargic or weak a lot of the time (and your doctor determines you're not sick), you could swap your after-meal siesta with an activity. Somewhat frustratingly, you'll find that the benefits of regular exercise are just as satisfying as a ten- or fifteen-minute nap.

I Don't Believe in Change

You like your morning playlist in alphabetical order, your coffee with two creams and one sugar, and your eggs over-medium. There's no need to deviate from that or any other of your regular routines, even in the face of professional advice, like "Hey, you should maybe replace the eggs because your cholesterol is a little high." Who does that doctor think she is, anyhow?

So what if people joke that you're set in your ways? Ways are awesome. Parkway, freeway, spillway, jetway, entryway, raceway—all fantastic ways. No, you have a specific method, and you like it. It's how you can focus on the important things like learning TikTok dances and catching up on that new cooking competition show.

Pretty Sure You're Fine . . .

Hey, pal, calm down. No one's saying you need to change anything . . . except maybe your doctor. Though, if your doctor says you need to change your diet or add exercise or anything else like that, you should listen because, as mentioned earlier in this book, they went to medical school.

You should also consider research conducted by the University of Southern California's Department of Psychology, which found non-necessary routines could be less about organization and more about habit and risk-aversion. And Kathleen Smith, PhD, suggests an inability or unwillingness to adapt to change can be detrimental. She writes, "If you can't cope with change, only a minor amount of stress can make you feel overwhelmed by life." And if that quote overwhelms you, you might need to make a change.

Change doesn't have to be drastic.

But here's why you're probably fine: Change doesn't have to be drastic. An adjustment in your diet (such as the preceding cholesterol example) could be as simple as switching from regular ol' eggs to egg whites. Adding exercise can be as easy as adding a few reps of burpees to your day. Making changes in small increments can have a huge effect without causing anxiety or stress. Besides, changing your routine can even boost your focus, creativity, and memory. So, maybe don't fear change so much. It could even be your superpower. Not as cool as laser eyes, but still.

Be Optimistic about Optimism

If you're feeling pessimistic because of, y'know, everything sucking all the time, you might want to try changing your outlook. Optimistic people live longer and healthier than Negative Nellies. They even have better cardiovascular health. That's generally because they make better decisions about their health. Who knows? You may also drive away annoying people with your positivity, so that's a bonus.

I'm Better at Telling Others What to Do

At lunch, you suggest to your friend that they might enjoy the shrimp quinoa instead of the steak sandwich. You cleverly framed it as a mere flavor issue, but added that the former has a lower calorie count, which was your true intent. Later, when chatting with your sister, you suggest she handle the emotional strain of raising twins with a little mindful meditation (you respectfully refrain from suggesting it was her fault for having twins in the first place). She always looked up to you, after all, and that's for a good reason: You can easily spot how other people can improve their life.

Your coworker feels rundown, so you suggest they swap that third cup of coffee for a short exercise routine. Your mailman tweaked his back, so you float the idea of low-impact stretches to keep that muscle limber and strong. Your neighbor feels overworked, so you pose that allowing just ten minutes of quiet "me time" daily could help reduce stress.

If only there was someone like that for you, someone who could clearly see the flaws in your life and how to address them. Alas, you'll just go on living as the stressed-out, unhealthy wreck of a human who can help others.

Pretty Sure You're Fine . . .

It's like your home is on fire and you're standing there with a hose going, "I wish someone could put out this fire." You. Have. The. HOSE!

Sure, it's hard to fix your own issues, but that's not your fault. Often, it's difficult to see solutions (or even problems) when we're looking inward. As communications and marketing expert Elissa Bertot writes, "When you're so close to your problem, you simply can't see it for what it is." She suggests you try turning the good advice you'd give others on yourself.

And a pair of 2019 surveys posed the question: "What advice would you give your younger self?" More than 50 percent of those who participated said they now take that advice.

So, whether you need to step back or time travel, you likely already know what steps you can take to improve your health and wellness. Time to start caring about yourself, pal. Okay? Okay. Now, who needs a hug?

Trick Yourself Healthy

Sometimes (okay, all of the time), rather than exercise, it seems more appealing to just eat tortilla chips from the bag while binging *Real Housewives of . . .* anywhere. Thank goodness science discovered ways to motivate yourself. One way is to give yourself a real reward, so not a well-earned sense of superiority, but, maybe a smoothie. Another motivator is finding a group of actual motivators. A group of buddies can motivate you in ways that guilt (or as one study found out, even gift cards) can't.

Nothing Matters, Anyway

Melting polar ice caps, mutating viruses, record heat waves, dating-show competitions, lactose intolerance—there's no point of caring about your health if this is what the world has to offer. Like, have you seen the lineup at Coachella? I mean, really.

You were thinking about getting in shape, losing a few pounds, just for the sake of your health, but now you're realizing we're all going to die in some embarrassing and stupid way, and you might as well be enjoying some Flamin' Hot Cheetos while it happens.

Pretty Sure You're Fine . . .

No, sure. I mean, you're right. Watching the news makes it seem like we could all die as early as Thursday. If that's your true outlook (and not just laziness), enjoy your final days. And allow me to offer a jaunty tip o' the hat to your commitment to this vague final timeline for all of humanity. In the shadow of a city-sized meteor racing toward Earth, yeah, pretty sure you're fine because "fine" in this case is relative and everyone in the scenario is screwed, so it's kind of an easy win, though seconds before your unavoidable flaming death.

And while those world-ending disasters are actually further off than you think, you might assume this section will pose a glass half-empty/half-full sort of philosophical attaboy in which I tell you that life's totally worth living healthily because of daisies and Pomeranian puppies and waterslides and Jamba Juice, but that's not going to happen. Instead, I'm going to ask a simple question: Do you want to be unhealthy at the exact moment when you'll need to be as healthy as possible?

Because when the giant multidimensional space aliens start rounding up us lowly humans for food and sport, you don't want to be the guy giving away your location by wheezing like an old water heater as you flee the invading horde. Yes, I suggest you care about your health simply to outrun or outlast whatever disaster will inevitably destroy us all. Molten lava moves pretty slow, but it moves faster than the guy who's solely ingested Froot Loops and Jägermeister for the past nine months. And it only takes a few weeks to fall out of shape when you stop exercising.

Molten lava moves pretty slow, but not as slow as the guy who's solely ingested Froot Loops and Jägermeister for the past nine months.

Of course, that feeling of "why does it matter?" is very common, especially when the news as of late has been pretty dire. Experts suggest you shake that feeling by focusing on how you felt when things were better. But, y'know, only if you want to.

WORKING
STIFF

I Love Work More Than I Love My Kids

You come home from work and your kids immediately smother you with their take on the latest *Fortnite* update or wave their phone in front of your face so you can see the meme their classmate made using a photo of a blobfish. All you want to do is sit in the recliner for five uninterrupted minutes and stare blissfully at the wall, but they just won't leave you alone.

You long for the peace, order, and quiet of the office. Your coworkers don't ask for help finding their shoes, which are right where they left them yesterday. They don't ask for a tuna sandwich and then not eat any of it. They don't get into an argument with their sibling about whether a common housecat could jump over a Fiat 500X.

With horror, you realize you enjoy being at your workplace more than at home with your chatty, energetic, feral offspring. And that makes you the worst parent who ever lived.

Pretty Sure You're Fine...

Shifting from one situation that demands all your attention to a totally different one that also demands all your attention can give you emotional and mental whiplash. It's perfectly common to have a rough re-entry from work each day, which could lead to pining for the comparatively mundane routine of your office. And there's a really good reason for that: No matter how challenging your job is, parenting is likely more stressful and physically demanding.

But don't mistake longing for a moment of respite for *not* loving your kids. Just because your children annoy you upon arrival, that doesn't make you a bad parent. It makes you a regular parent. Like, totally, super, incredibly regular.

Just because your children annoy you upon arrival, that doesn't make you a bad parent.

To ease the transition from work to home, you should find a way to definitively separate them. The simplest way is to make your commute a sort of meditation—listen to calming music or no music (mindful driving?). Another thing to try is forcing yourself to take a small personal break before jumping back into your parenting duties, like enjoying a cup o' joe at a coffee shop before heading home, doing a short workout, sitting in the park to read for fifteen minutes, or—I don't know—strapping on a utility belt and fighting crime. So, give yourself a break, figuratively and literally.

I'm Bored
at Work

Thankfully, you have high cubicle walls because if they were just a bit shorter your coworkers and manager would see that you've reached the "Card Shark" level on your solitaire app, and that you've amassed quite a following on TikTok, where you demonstrate semiweekly how to make entertaining mechanisms out of basic office supplies. So far no one in your office seems to notice that you go through paper clips awful rapidly for a person who doesn't print much. And these activities are barely enough to keep you from dozing off on your keyboard.

You fear someday your boss will come around the corner and see you celebrating your latest victory in *Among Us* or your nosy officemate will rat you out for making an armada of little battleships out of Post-it Notes. But what could possibly be done? There's simply not that much work to do and the work you do have is *sooooooooo boring*. You're not sure if this counts as stealing, but it's not your fault the company is so poorly run that they don't realize you're using company time to become a social media influencer.

Pretty Sure You're Fine . . .

This may sound weird, but an article in *Psychology Today* suggests your boredom is not necessarily bad. And you're not alone. Apparently, 30 to 90 percent of adults feel bored. That's quite a spread, and it means you could use one of those office supply mechanisms to launch a rubber band ball at random in your office and you'd likely hit a coworker who's also bored out of their skull. So, yeah, you're good.

But, if you want to cure that boredom, the article also states: "Boredom can be a catalyst for action." And it's a great opportunity to take some initiative with a work project or bring your—*ahem*—free time to your manager's attention to see if there's a way to utilize your skills or even learn new ones. You could also try setting some of your own personal goals or assign yourself a project.

Of course, being bored at work could mean you are in the wrong vocation or you're not being challenged. So another action you could take is to use your downtime at work to look for a job that excites you more . . . hey, maybe the paper clip factory is hiring! Or

Hey, maybe the paper clip factory is hiring!

you can really shake things up with something super-drastic, like dangling from a helicopter while wearing a panda costume that is also on fire (though, that's not recommended by any sane professional with the exception of the Helicopter-Dangling Flaming Cosplay Association, which is a totally made-up thing. So, seriously, don't do that.).

I'm Incompetent at My Job

Your boss tasked you with opening up the shop on Saturday. You smiled and thanked her for the opportunity to show your potential. As soon as she turned to walk back to the office, however, your face fell into a terrified frown. You don't even know where the keys to the shop door are kept. Probably a drawer of some kind? Maybe a hook?

As your boss gathers her things to leave, panic sets into your bones so powerfully you have an uncontrolled moment of astral projection in which your soul leaves your body and travels into the future—a future in which you totally blow the shop opening and get fired in front of a crowd of angry customers and TV news cameras that are on the scene for some reason, and then you're left penniless and perpetually couch-surfing until you can land your next job from which you'll also get fired.

Pretty Sure You're Fine . . .
Your boss would not have given you this particular assignment if she didn't think you could handle it. And lots of people feel like they're not up to the challenge when given more responsibility, even when that responsibility comes in the form of writing a book on

110

stress-free ways to improve your health and wellness . . . *cough, cough.*

Anyway, there are a few stress-free ways to deal with that self-doubt, like acknowledging your self-doubt, realizing everyone makes mistakes (if you even do make any), and that you can actually talk to your boss about your concerns. Who'd have thought asking your boss for tips on completing the task she assigned you might be a smart thing to do? Crazy, huh? And almost no boss will be upset when asked for work advice. That's basically what they're there for. That, and looking at spreadsheets while they make low grunts of what may be comprehension.

Your insecurities or fears about failing may actually mean you're a perfectionist, which isn't a terrible thing.

Also, your insecurities or fears about failing may actually mean you're a perfectionist, which isn't a terrible thing. Many wildly successful people such as Elon Musk, Serena Williams, and Gordon Ramsay confess that they're perfectionists who also grapple with the looming and near-constant fear of failure.

You'll do fine. No, you'll do great. Just make sure the TV news crew gets your good side.

My Work Stresses Me Out

You arrive at work and your teeth clench so tight you could bite down on a chunk of coal and make a diamond. As the morning goes on, your muscles feel sore from all the tension stored in them, and you can't even justify it by blaming it on a good workout. You check the daily schedule and see what's up next: staff meeting. Your stomach feels ill and not the fun kind of ill you get while riding a roller coaster or doing too many shots of honey-infused whiskey.

And there's no respite. On the commute home, you think about projects and reports left to finish and coworkers' lame dating stories to sit through during lunch. At home, you can't relax because you know in just twelve hours or so you're going to be right back in that gaping hellhole of screaming lost souls called an office.

You try to sleep, but your body refuses and decides instead to do a mental recap of what happened that day and a forecast of what you have to look forward to tomorrow. It's like a mental trapeze act swinging from one stressful situation to the other, without a net, without a harness, and without dental coverage. At least there are snacks in the break room.

Pretty Sure You're Fine . . .

If you can't stop stressing about your job, there's nothing really wrong with you. A lot of people experience work-related stress. Like, seriously, a *lot*. A Northwestern National Life survey found that 40 percent of workers said their job was "very or extremely stressful." And that stress can come from many different places, whether financial (low pay), or professional (no ladder or an unrealistically heavy workload), or personal (you're just bored out of your damned mind).

Needless to say (but here it is, anyway), that kind of prolonged stress can do some real mental and physical harm. So while you're not alone, you should take some action. Learning how to manage and mitigate stress will do the most good because, quite frankly, even the most fun jobs in the world are still stressful now and again. Just ask a carny—seems like a blast, but their work isn't all fun and games. . . . Well, it is fun and games, but . . . I mean . . . you know.

Do You Even Woodwork, Bro?

Lots of people look forward to the moment when they can leave work and head to the gym. But what is an employee to do when their gym shuts down due to a kaiju attack or a Biblical flood or, say, a pandemic?

At the beginning of the 2020 pandemic, former Army police officer Zachary Skidmore of Jackson, Ohio, lamented the temporary shutdown of his local gym. When he eyed a fallen tree on his property, however, he felt a flash of inspiration. And, as any jacked, ex-military, exercise enthusiast with a chainsaw would do, he constructed an entire gym's worth of workout equipment—shoulder press, leg press, weights, even a treadmill—out of wood. Sure, the result is admirable, but the splinters are hell.

My Boss
Is Out to
Get Me

You first noticed it in a company meeting—the stern glance from across the room. At first you chalked it up to misreading the look on his face, but your boss doesn't often throw stern glances. The next time you noticed it was at the watercooler when you asked him what he thought of last night's football game. He didn't even acknowledge you and just walked away.

These types of behaviors aren't unfamiliar to you. After all, you've had a couple of romantic relationships start to go south with these exact kinds of interactions. You can safely assume your boss isn't upset with you because you've neglected to bring him flowers, so what could it be? The fact that you don't always refill the coffeemaker? The scent of your deodorant? Your enviable charm?

He doesn't treat anyone else this way, so you come to the very logical conclusion that he just hates you. He's just waiting for the next missed memo or budget miscalculation to bring the axe down and send you out into the parking lot with your personal items stuffed in an old banker box.

Pretty Sure You're Fine...

The worst thing you can do in a situation like this is assume what your boss (or anyone who seems irrationally upset) thinks or feels about you. Unless you're one of a handful of comic book or horror movie characters, you can't read anyone's mind.

Unless you're one of a handful of comic book or horror movie characters, you can't read anyone's mind.

Plus, there are plenty of easy ways to discern if your boss is actually mad at you or is just having an off week. And, this may sound unreasonably simple, but the easiest way is because they'll tell you so. Yes, believe it or not, bosses will usually let you know if you're screwing up. That's why they have those chairs across from their desk, so they can lean on said desk, trap you in that chair with their gaze, and tell you how much you suck. It's one of the many perks of being in charge.

On the occasion that your boss does actually have an issue with you, that doesn't mean they hate you. Professional disagreements happen, and they might just be irked at the way you handled a problem or a task. The way to clarify all of this is to simply ask them if they're upset with you and, if so, how to remedy it. Yeah, it's awful how open communication solves everything.

My Employer Doesn't Care about Physical Health

You like your coworkers and your paycheck. Heck, you even like your workspace. But the company for which you work doesn't seem to like you. Or at least, they don't care whether or not you're healthy. (Perhaps you shouldn't have taken that extra ten minutes during lunch.)

The break room pantry is full of salty and sugary snacks, break times aren't long enough to fit in any kind of workout, and you can't even get up and move around unless you're heading to the bathroom. Your dastardly employer obviously wants you fat and tired so you can sit and do more work. The villainy!

Pretty Sure You're Fine . . .

The fact that you're concerned about your health at all is a huge advantage. Many people don't think about their health at work, a shame considering most people spend literally one-third of their life working. If your employer doesn't offer ways to maintain a healthy lifestyle at work, you have two options, one of which is completely in your control. Let's start with the latter.

Legally, you should have no fear raising your concerns to your boss or even HR. That doesn't mean they're obligated to switch to healthier snacks or offer exercise options, but at least it'll put it on their radar, especially if you can get a number of coworkers to lodge similar concerns. There is strength in numbers. Together you can win! Victory! Attica! I am Spartacus!

(If your issue involves an illness or injury, however, you should consult with your doctor about who needs to know and your employee handbook about any necessary disclosures, especially if any such health issue prevents you from doing the job for which you were hired. We now return to our regularly scheduled informational smartassery.)

The option that's completely in your control is to, well, take control.

The option that's completely in your control is to, y'know, take control. Bring your own healthy snacks and even though a fifteen-minute break may not seem like enough time to exercise, it totally is—walk around the building a few times, do pushups in the parking lot, jumping jacks in the vacant office down the hall, smash some board with your head, scale a tree. You can also do simple exercises at your desk, like calf raises and lunges. Even a small amount of exercise is better than no exercise.

These Fluorescent Lights Are Killing Me

You can feel it in the air, that numbing radiation . . . or maybe it's gamma rays or something. Those damn buzzing fluorescent lights in the office are slowly poisoning you while you work.

Sure, they seem so innocuous, so innocent. Like, "Oh, we're just happy little glowing tubes here to light your way and brighten your day." But you know the sinister truth. They're malicious Satan rods bent on ravaging your body with unseen waves of pure evil. If you concentrate, you can feel the tumors growing in your body, your organs systematically shutting down.

To the layperson, you sound paranoid, but you have proof. Yes, hard proof! Your eyes are sunken and your skin is pale. Your energy level feels as if you've just come from an all-night bender and you're fairly certain your hair is starting to fall out. Time to start a GoFundMe page to pay for your rapidly approaching funeral.

Pretty Sure You're Fine . . .

Despite all the rumors and "common knowledge," fluorescent lighting poses no harm to you, your coworkers, your desk plant, the bike messenger that shows up every Tuesday, or the sandwich cart guy.

Now, fluorescent lights do emit a bit of radiation, but less than your cell phone, and you're fine having that in your pocket all day. They can also exacerbate migraines, but only because migraine sufferers are more sensitive to light, anyway. Their "blue light" can disrupt your body's production of melatonin (the hormone that manages your body's sleep schedule), but only if you're sitting under or around them at bedtime. And, really, why would you ever do that?

Fluorescent lights do emit a bit of radiation, but less than your cell phone, and you're fine having that in your pocket all day.

That said, we're indoors a lot—80 to 90 percent of our time is spent in an office or other structure. And sunlight offers a lot of mental and physical benefits, such as a calming effect and vitamin D. In fact, a survey by Future Workplace revealed that workers covet natural light so much it topped the list of requested office perks. So, while the fluorescent lights aren't poisoning you, getting outside every once in a while wouldn't hurt. Neither would trimming that weird hair in your ears, but that's not relevant right now.

I'm Afraid It's Too Late to Report a Work-Related Injury

You rolled your ankle while moving some boxes. It was a bit embarrassing because you kind of squealed a bit and it sounded like a cheerleader who spotted a caterpillar in her garden salad wrap. You limped back to your desk to let it rest and later iced it at home because you've had similar injuries before and you don't need a doctor to tell you what basic common sense does.

But, after a week, your ankle still feels sore and unsteady. You find yourself favoring your other leg and your gait resembles the lead-in to a fabulous disco number. Now, your basic common sense has changed its tune from one of calm and cool self-care to a bellowing death metal ballad urging you to see a specialist. But you can't afford that, and you fear you may have missed your window to report it to your employer. Alas, you will simply live out the rest of your days with a limp that grows ever worse until you're forced to wheel yourself to and from the break room in your office chair.

Pretty Sure You're Fine . . .

Clearly, your ankle isn't fine, but when it comes to reporting your injury, yeah, you're likely okay. Most state laws make it possible to report a work-related

What A Tool

Think your job sucks? At least you weren't tasked with creating the next big fitness device only to see it become the unshapely butt of jokes. Here are a few of the greatest fitness product fails:

Sauna Suit: It looked like a jumpsuit made from garbage bags and claimed to help you lose weight fast by making you sweat like a teenage boy at a burlesque show.

ThighMaster: Despite celebrity Suzanne Somers lending her name and face to this device that looked like a giant bent paper clip, it never became a fitness revolution.

Shake Weight: The Big Weiner . . . I mean, the Big Winner of all horrifying fitness products, this special free weight made users looked like they were handling a penis . . . like, aggressively handling it.

injury as far out as thirty days from the incident, and some even provide a window of ninety days or longer. (There are a few that require you to report it "as soon as possible" or within three days—I'm looking at you, South Dakota—but those aren't the norm.)

In many work environments, you are *required* to report any injury, no matter how seemingly insignificant. Plus, if the potential treatment leads to exorbitant medical bills or if your employer was somehow at fault, you need to have a record of your experience. So, don't "walk it off" or "ride it out." You should not be walking or riding anything. As the old song goes: Billy, don't be a hero. And that applies to all people not named Billy as well.

NO
LAUGHING
MATTER

My Weight Affects My Health

Maybe you weren't paying attention, maybe you were but just didn't think it mattered, or maybe an underlying health issue played the key role, but you've gained some unwanted weight. And now it's affecting things other than your clothing size.

Your energy level has tanked, your self-esteem remains low, and your doctor is concerned about cholesterol, heart disease, diabetes . . . everything. But you feel like you're too far gone at this point. There's no way to ever recover from this state and this weight. Like biological Whac-A-Mole, you'll just have to deal with those related health issues as they come.

Pretty Sure You Can Be Fine . . .

There's no easy way to say this: You have to do something. Sure, a doctor can provide guidance and advice, prescriptions, and referrals for other doctors, but ultimately the motivation part is up to you. You need to be the one that cares about yourself and your health.

And listen, everybody's body is different, but you know yours. You know what you can do. So, if your doctor says you need to lose weight, don't throw up your hands. Start small. The benefits of a simple walk have been mentioned many times in this book. Here's one benefit that hasn't been mentioned much: Because it's low impact (easy on the joints), walking is ideal for people who are overweight and obese.

Experts advise overweight individuals to get thirty minutes of exercise a day. That may sound daunting, but if broken up into three ten-minute walks, it's easier to hit that goal. And an article on Healthline suggests you "don't allow yourself to get hung up on the clock. Instead, focus on picking an activity that you enjoy and that can fit into your schedule at least three to five days a week." (This advice also appears earlier in the book, which you'd know if you didn't skip around with no regard for page numbers or basic book structure.)

There's no easy way to say this: You have to do something.

And if there's an underlying condition affecting your weight, like thyroid or kidney issues, talk to your doctor about what you can and should do in conjunction with whatever medical treatment they suggest. And, hey, you can do this, okay?

I Suffered a Debilitating Injury and Need Physical Therapy

You prepared for every possible health eventuality. You have a strict regimen of vitamins, whole foods, and exercise. When it comes to your own wellness, you are an Adonis . . . until that one tumble. Or maybe it was an accident. Or maybe it was just a part of your dumb body bending the wrong dumb way.

It shouldn't have been as bad as it was. A simple misstep around the coffee table and now your arm (or leg or back) is wrecked and your planned summer of swimming parties are all as busted as your body.

What, you wonder, was the point of staying so healthy if your body was just going to crap out anyway? You contemplate the monotony of needed physical recovery and decide it's time to see why everyone's always raving about Burger King. If your body doesn't care, there's no reason you should either.

Pretty Sure You Can Be Fine . . .

Do you know why the old saying goes "accidents happen?" Because they do. And yeah, it sucks that you take great care of yourself or at least try to be careful and yet injuries feel like they wipe out all of that away.

Don't let the injury get you down. In fact, in this moment self-care is more important than ever. Because, depending on the injury, you may need to level up that self-care to prevent long-term health effects down the road. Yeah, we're talking about physical therapy.

If your physician recommends physical therapy, you'll learn for some types of injuries physical therapy can be at the least tiresome and annoying and at its worst downright painful, but you really should do it, no matter what. The alternative could land anywhere between reduced functionality and complete loss of motor function.

And hey, in some cases, physical therapy can speed recovery and even reduce the need for surgery. So, be your own hero. You'll be back to those swimming parties in no time.

Level up that self-care to prevent long-term health effects down the road.

I Have a Bad Habit That Affects Me and Others

The nightly cocktail you employed to unwind after work became two, then three. Before you knew it, you were blowing through bottles faster than teenagers at a backyard shooting gallery. You started sleeping later to make up for the restless nights that followed, which made you show up late for work. Now, your projects are suffering and your coworkers can't trust you. Or maybe it was something else—a pill to ease your pain that grew into a daily routine, or a string of self-destructive physical relationships.

You see the pattern and you know its unhealthy, so you tried to stop, to quell the behavior and get yourself back on track. But when you promise yourself that you'll keep it to one drink or one pill or one night of fun, the floodgates open again and you're back in the same old self-destructive routine, except now you also feel like a failure for not being able to keep your indulgences in check. You decide it's better to just roll with your habit for now. Maybe you can try to change things next week.

Pretty Sure You Can Be Fine . . .

This isn't just a habit, it's likely an addiction. You probably know some of the usual signs of addiction such as reverting to harmful behaviors or anxiousness over the thought of stopping, but the easiest one to recognize is "lack of control, or inability to stay away from a substance or behavior." If this hits home for you, there are plenty of ways and places to get help, such as 12-step programs, rational emotive behavior therapy, and contingency management.

Of course, taking that first step—actually seeking help—is often the hardest part. But it's also the most freeing and powerful part because it's you taking control and committing to begin the work to better yourself.

While you can recover, you shouldn't attempt to do it alone.

While you can recover, you shouldn't attempt to do it alone. Lean on a friend or reach out to a medical professional and make a plan. And know that you can do this. Your recovery *is* possible.

Mental Health (Finally) Takes Center Stage

For decades, experts have called for a destigmatizing of mental health issues and recently this effort picked up a star-studded head of steam due in large part to celebrities such as Chrissy Teigen and Dwayne Johnson sharing their stories and truthful depictions of mental health in shows and films. Now, experts are offering advice on how employers can help their employees improve and maintain their mental health.

I Don't Have Health Insurance

You never saw the need for health insurance and things have gone swimmingly so far. You're pretty healthy, you exercise regularly, you don't do drugs, and you're young. You won't go so far as to say you're never going to die, but Death's going to have to come at you with an arsenal and a posse to take you down at some ripe old age.

If your employer offered it, sure, you'd sign up. But they don't, so you make sure you have echinacea and vitamins on hand and look both ways before crossing the street. If something does happen that requires more medical attention, you're sure you can figure it out. After all, what's the worst that can happen?

Pretty Sure You Can Be Fine . . .

Dude, get health coverage.

You can't ride on luck forever and when (not if, *when*) you need medical care, aside from whatever injury or illness with which you must grapple, it will destroy your bank account. Yes, it will wreak more financial havoc than the cost of getting health coverage. University of Maryland School of Public Health's Associate Professor of the Health Services Administration, Dylan Roby, says, "A cancer diagnosis, car accident, or even a broken leg can cost thousands of dollars out-of-pocket." In fact, two-thirds of those who file for bankruptcy cite medical costs as the main factor.

But, hey, there's good news. If you're unemployed, can't get coverage through work, or can't find an inexpensive option from an insurance company, thanks to the Affordable Care Act and other programs (a.k.a the Marketplace), there are a handful of low- or no-cost options, such as Medicaid or the Children's Health Insurance Program. Also, recently increased funding for local medical clinics makes it easier for people to get the care they need. So, just do it.

Worry Yourself Healthy

All the best wellness plans include deep meditative stuff like "letting go of negative emotions." So you might assume that includes worry, because worry often brings unnecessary stress and anxiety. But according to research, worrying may actually provide some benefits.

While too much worry can lead to "depressed mood, poor physical health, and even mental illness," many professionals also agree that the right amount of the right kind of worry can help motivate you and even protect you emotionally. And don't worry that you're worrying incorrectly. Here's a smart person to explain it.

University of Denver professor and worryologist (I just made up that word) Shelly Smith-Acuña, PhD, says, "Adaptive worry alerts you to dangers and threats, clarifies the problem, can lead you to seek help or more information from others, and then helps you solve the problem."

Basically, people who experience adaptive worry about a health concern are more likely to seek out professional help to address it. Similarly, those who worry about an unpleasant work situation or bad relationship tend to fix it or move on faster. So, in those cases, do *not* be chill. Go ahead and worry away.

I'm Depressed

Your job lost its luster years ago and now your shift does nothing but numb your brain. Not even your coworker's stories of their disastrous dating life lift your spirits. You zone out until bedtime and don't even remember what you did or what chores you were supposed to do. And then, in bed, you stare at the ceiling, unable to sleep because your body and brain simply aren't tired. Or sometimes, it feels more like you're *too* tired to sleep. And when you do sleep, you don't want to get out of bed in the morning. At all.

This is the cycle you trudge through each day and suffer through each night. The few occasional moments of happiness, joy, or even just what you assume is normalcy that you experience are fleeting at best, quickly swallowed up by the ever-looming melancholy. Is this it? Is this what life is supposed to be, just a series of repeated soulless experiences until retirement?

Pretty Sure You Can Be Fine . . .

It may not make a difference to you right now, but you're not alone. According to the World Health Organization, "more than 264 million people of all ages suffer from depression." This next piece of information, however, should make a difference: This is not your fault, but it's up to you to take the first step in dealing with it.

Now, you can probably guess some of the suggested methods for coping with depression: Eat healthy, get plenty of sleep, exercise. But the horrible truth is that, for people with depression, those things are seemingly the hardest to do. Yeah, so, you're not wrong. It sucks. A lot.

That's why you should also consider seeing a mental health professional. As stated earlier in this very book, seeking professional help *is* self-care. You can check with your insurer to see which therapists are covered, ask your physician for a referral, or just see if a friend or two can recommend someone. And when you do find a professional, child and adolescent psychotherapist Katie Hurley, LCSW, suggests you first ask questions about their experience and methods, and whether or not they can prescribe medications (if needed).

Also, take this as an opportunity to re-address and revamp your life. Who do you want to be? What do you want to do? Turn that into a plan with goals and get started.

Final Perspective

Y'know, there's a reason people say they feel bad after binge-eating a whole tub of ice cream, and it ain't lactose intolerance. Well, not always. It's guilt with a dash of shame and a light sprinkling of disappointment. For most of us, we already know what to do about our health concerns or . . . let's call them "not-so-great choices." Of course, actually implementing changes to improve our mental or physical health (or both) often feels like an overwhelming task and that's because making drastic changes in our lives seems—no, *is*—incredibly daunting. Like, super daunting. There are tons and tons of daunt there.

Hopefully, you've realized by this point what this whole book has been about. If not, here you go in plain ol' language: You deserve to be healthy, and chances are you already know what needs to be done to achieve that. However, it doesn't take a major overhaul of your life to do this. It takes only that first step toward a healthier you. Then, when you're ready, the next step. Then, the next. Then, the next and, hey, look! You're walking! Who's a big boy? Who's my big boy?

One other thing to keep in mind is that everybody struggles. Everybody. Even your friend with the perfect body and permanent smile is likely going through some heavy stuff, and that smile might act as a mask so she can avoid awkward conversations about it.

Things are likely not as dire as you might think they are.

And really, it's none of your business, anyway, Mr. Curious McNosy. So, no matter what you're going through, know you're not alone.

Finally, please, be kind to yourself. Forgive yourself. Because things are likely not as dire as you might think they are. Just make a commitment to yourself and look at whatever change you face not as a challenge, but as a gift you're giving yourself. And when it comes to your well-being, there are no dead ends and there is no limit to the number of attempts to improve yourself and your health, even if you've just finished off that pint of Dreyer's Butter Pecan. Or to put it in another, more succinct way . . .

Pretty Sure You're Fine.

Sources

"Lego-Plastic Fricken Lego Bricks," My Fitness Pal, https://www.myfitnesspal.com/food/calories/plastic-fricken-lego-bricks-184383508.

Peter Moore, "Two-fifths of Americans Are Tired Most of the Week," YouGovAmerica, https://today.yougov.com/topics/lifestyle/articles-reports/2015/06/02/sleep-and-dreams.

"Exercising for Better Sleep," Johns Hopkins Medicine, https://www.hopkinsmedicine.org/health/wellness-and-prevention/exercising-for-better-sleep.

Diana Rodriguez, "Why Exercise Boosts Mood and Energy," *Everyday Health*, https://www.everydayhealth.com/fitness/workouts/boost-your-energy-level-with-exercise.aspx.

"Why Your Metabolism Slows Down with Age," Healthline, https://www.healthline.com/nutrition/metabolism-and-age.

"Not Seeing Results? Five Common Weight Loss Methods that Might be Sabotaging Your Progress," Fitness Blender, https://www.fitnessblender.com/articles/not-seeing-results-5-common-weight-loss-methods-that-might-be-sabotaging-your-progress.

Kris Gunnars, BSc, "20 Common Reasons Why You're Not Losing as Much Weight as You Expected To," Healthline, https://www.healthline.com/nutrition/20-reasons-you-are-not-losing-weight.

Rina Deshpande, "Yoga in America Often Exploits My Culture—but You May Not Even Realize It," *Self*, https://www.self.com/story/yoga-indian-cultural-appropriation.

William Kremer, "Does Doing Yoga Make You a Hindu?," BBC News, https://www.bbc.com/news/magazine-25006926.

Megan Holstein, "Western Yoga is a Great Example of Cultural Appropriation," https://meganholstein.medium.com/western-yoga-is-a-great-example-of-cultural-appropriation-5d2f721b18c0.

Activif Team, "12 Compelling Alternatives to Yoga (Expand Your Horizons!)," Activif, https://www.activif.com/12-compelling-alternatives-to-yoga-expand-your-horizons/

Cory Stieg, "Do You Pass Gas in Yoga Class? You're Not Alone," Refinery29, June 3, 2019, https://www.refinery29.com/en-us/why-yoga-fart.

Roxy Menzies, "Core Galore: 15 Pilates Exercises to Develop Your Powerhouse," Healthline, April 26, 2021, https://www.healthline.com/health/fitness/pilates-exercises#what-is-pilates.

Agnes Nagy, "Callanetics® - Superb Exercise Programme based upon Ballet and Yoga," Positive Health Online, March, 2009 http://www.positivehealth.com/article/bodywork/callanetics-r-superb-exercise-programme-based-upon-ballet-and-yoga.

Lydia House and Morgan Fargo, "12 Major Benefits of Swimming You NTK: From Muscle Building to Injury Rehab," *Women's Health*, Feb. 16, 2021, https://www.womenshealthmag.com/uk/fitness/g27268961/benefits-of-swimming/.

Richie Allen, "Jack LaLanne Workout," Muscle Prodigy, https://www.muscleprodigy.com/jack-lalanne-workout/.

Christa Sgobba, CPT, "A Fun and Simple Beginner Workout at Home without Equipment," Self, January 9, 2021, https://www.self.com/gallery/beginner-workout-at-home-with-no-equipment.

Dr. Ty E. Richardson, "Orthopedic Warning: Beware of Boot Camp Fitness Classes," New Mexico Orthopedics, July 3, 2018, https://www.nmortho.com/orthopedic-warning-beware-of-boot-camp-fitness-classes/.

"Boot Camp Workout: Is It Right for You?," Mayo Clinic, https://www.mayoclinic.org/healthy-lifestyle/fitness/in-depth/boot-camp-workout/art-20046363.

"How the Mainstream Media Is Destroying Your Body Image," *The Active Times*, September 23, 2014, https://www.theactivetimes.com/how-mainstream-media-destroying-your-body-image.

Neil Farber, MD, PhD, "It's Not Your Fault - Blame Biology!," *Psychology Today*, September 7, 2010, https://www.psychologytoday.com/us/blog/the-blame-game/201009/its-not-your-fault-blame-biology.

Emily DiNuzzo, "A Victoria's Secret Model Trainer Reveals Why You Should Never Try to Work Out Like an Angel," *Insider*, September 5, 2017, https://www.insider.com/personal-trainer-victorias-secret-models-body-image-2017-9.

"3 Reasons to Work Out With a Friend," Centers for Disease Control and Prevention, https://www.cdc.gov/diabetes/library/spotlights/workout-buddy.html.

"The Health Benefits of Working Out with a Crowd," NBC News, https://www.nbcnews.com/better/health/why-you-should-work-out-crowd-ncna798936.

Jane Chertoff, "Does Sweating Help You Burn More Calories?," Healthline, updated September 18, 2018, https://www.healthline.com/health/does-sweating-burn-calories.

Carina Wolff, "Try These Exercises If You Hate Sweating," Bustle, November 23, 2015, https://www.bustle.com/articles/125458-7-exercises-if-you-hate-sweating-because-you-can-work-out-without-overheating.

Elizabeth Narins, "9 Tricks to Get Fit without Getting All Sweaty," Cosmopolitan, October 10. 2016, https://www.cosmopolitan.com/health-fitness/a5083945/workout-tricks-that-dont-make-you-sweat/.

Cory Stieg, "Do You Pass Gas in Yoga Class? You're Not Alone," Refinery29, June 3, 2019, https://www.refinery29.com/en-us/why-yoga-fart.

Mercey Livingston, "The Most Effective Workouts to Get in Shape in the Least Amount of Time," CNET, December 28, 2019, https://www.cnet.com/health/fitness/the-most-effective-workouts-to-get-in-shape-in-the-least-amount-of-time/.

Paige Waehner, "12 Time-Efficient and Effective Exercises You're Not Doing," Verywell Fit, October 30, 2020, https://www.verywellfit.com/time-efficient-effective-exercises-4101809.

Jade Poole, "What Is the Difference between Cardio and Strength Training?,"MyMed.com, https://www.mymed.com/health-wellness/fitness-and-exercise/the-case-of-cardio-cracked/what-is-the-difference-between-cardio-and-strength-training.

"How to Meditate: 5 Meditation Tips for Beginners," MasterClass, updated March 3, 2021, https://www.masterclass.com/articles/how-to-meditate#5-meditation-tips-for-beginners.

"What Is Mindfulness?," University of Minnesota Earl E. Bakken Center for Spirituality & Healing, https://www.takingcharge.csh.umn.edu/what-mindfulness.

Emma Seppala, PhD, "An Incredible Alternative to Mindfulness You Never Heard of," Psychology Today, April 19, 2016, https://www.psychologytoday.com/us/blog/feeling-it/201604/incredible-alternative-mindfulness-you-never-heard.

"Stress Relievers: Tips to Tame Stress," Mayo Clinic, https://www.mayoclinic.org/healthy-lifestyle/stress-management/in-depth/stress-relievers/art-20047257.

Kristeen Cherney, "Therapies That Work for Stress," Healthline, November 3, 2020, https://www.healthline.com/health/therapy-for-stress#therapies-for-stress.

Wendy Miller, "Fall Asleep during Meditation? Try These 12 Tips!," Start It Up, June 6, 2019, https://medium.com/swlh/fall-asleep-during-meditation-try-these-12-tips-6f018ee255bc.

"How Many Hours of Sleep Are Enough for Good Health?," Mayo Clinic, https://www.mayoclinic.org/healthy-lifestyle/adult-health/expert-answers/how-many-hours-of-sleep-are-enough/faq-20057898.

Elizabeth Beasley, "Best Hobbies for Mental Health," Healthgrades, https://www.healthgrades.com/right-care/mental-health-and-behavior/best-hobbies-for-mental-health.

"The Science behind Why Hobbies Can Improve Our Mental Health," The Conversation, February 11, 2021, https://theconversation.com/the-science-behind-why-hobbies-can-improve-our-mental-health-153828.

"Fixed-Effects Analyses of Time-Varying Associations between Hobbies and Depression in a Longitudinal Cohort Study: Support for Social Prescribing?," Karger International, https://www.karger.com/Article/FullText/503571.

Jessica Grace, "Therapy Isn't Something to Be Ashamed of," The Gottman Institute, March 13, 2018, https://www.gottman.com/blog/therapy-isnt-something-ashamed/.

Maggie Marshall, "Why I Chose to Seek Counseling," GenTwenty, December 26, 2014, https://gentwenty.com/chose-seek-counseling/.

"Cannabidiol as a Potential Treatment for Anxiety Disorders," PMC Neurotherapeutics, https://www.ncbi.nlm.nih.gov/pmc/articles/PMC4604171/.

Dennis Thompson, "More Are Turning to Pot When Depressed–But Does It Help or Harm?," WebMD, September 10, 2020, https://www.webmd.com/depression/news/20200910/more-are-turning-to-pot-when-depressed--but-does-it-help-or-harm.

Ziba Kashef, "Beta Blockers Reduce Stress-Induced Irregular Heart Rhythm," YaleNews, June 4, 2019, https://news.yale.edu/2019/06/04/beta-blockers-reduce-stress-induced-irregular-heart-rhythm.

Abigail Brenner, MD, "5 Benefits of Stepping Outside Your Comfort Zone," *Psychology Today*, December 27, 2015, https://www.psychologytoday.com/us/blog/in-flux/201512/5-benefits-stepping-outside-your-comfort-zone.

Steven Novella, "Mindfulness No Better Than Watching TV," *Neurologica*, February 6, 2018, https://theness.com/neurologicablog/index.php/mindfulness-no-better-than-watching-tv/.

Meghan Neal, "Is Watching TV Actually a Good Way to Rest Your Brain?," Vice, January 18, 2016, https://www.vice.com/en/article/3daqaj/is-watching-tv-actually-a-good-way-to-rest-your-brain.

Alexandra Sifferlin, "Watching TV to Relieve Stress Can Make You Feel Like a Failure," *Time*, July 24, 2014, https://time.com/3029797/watching-tv-to-relieve-stress-can-make-you-feel-like-a-failure/.

Amir Khan, "7 Ways Pets Can Make You Healthier," *U.S. News & World Report*, July 25, 2014, https://health.usnews.com/health-news/health-wellness/slideshows/7-ways-pets-can-make-you-healthier.

"Five Ways Pets Make Our Lives Better," Lifespan, August 29, 2019, https://www.lifespan.org/lifespan-living/five-ways-pets-make-our-lives-better.

Giang Cao Ho My, MA, "What Are the Origins of Mindfulness," *Thrive Global*, November 30, 2020, https://thriveglobal.com/stories/what-are-the-origins-of-mindfulness/.

Andres Fossas, "The Basics of Mindfulness: Where Did It Come From?," *WellDoing.org*, January 27, 2015, https://welldoing.org/article/basics-of-mindfulness-come-from.

Christina Sciarrillo, Jillian Joyce, Deana Hildebrand, and Sam Emerson, "The Health Risks of Fad Diets," Oklahoma State University: Extension, November 2020, https://extension.okstate.edu/fact-sheets/the-health-risk-of-fad-diets.html.

Kris Gunnars BSc, "20 Common Reasons Why You're Not Losing as Much Weight as You Expected To," Healthline, updated June 15, 2021, https://www.healthline.com/nutrition/20-reasons-you-are-not-losing-weight.

Grant Stoddard, "27 Things a Juice Cleanse Does to Your Body," Eat This, Not That!, December 29, 2015, https://www.eatthis.com/juice-cleanse-effects/.

Lauren Cooper, "Is a Juice Cleanse Right for You?," Consumer Reports, January 27, 2016, https://www.consumerreports.org/diet-nutrition/is-a-juice-cleanse-right-for-you/.

Jane Chertoff, "19 High-Protein Vegetables and How to Eat More of Them," Healthline, updated August 20, 2019, https://www.healthline.com/health/food-nutrition/19-high-protein-vegetables.

Elaine Howley, "Pescatarian vs. Vegetarian," *U.S. News & World Report*, November 25, 2019, https://health.usnews.com/wellness/compare-diets/articles/pescatarian-vs-vegetarian.

"Here's the Deal with Your Junk Food Cravings," Cleveland Clinic, December 14, 2020, https://health.clevelandclinic.org/heres-the-deal-with-your-junk-food-cravings/.

"Beat Your Cravings: 8 Effective Techniques," The Mayo Clinic Diet, https://diet.mayoclinic.org/diet/eat/beat-your-cravings.

Diane Carbonell, "The Big Picture: A Weekly Calorie Allowance," HealthWay, November 17, 2015, https://www.healthyway.com/content/the-big-picture-a-weekly-calorie-allowance/.

Wendy Bumgardner, "How Many Calories Do You Burn Walking Per Mile?," Verywell Fit, updated December 12, 2019, https://www.verywellfit.com/walking-calories-burned-by-miles-3887154.

Joel Furhman, MD, "The Hidden Dangers of Fast and Processed Food," *American Journal of Lifestyle Medicine*, https://www.ncbi.nlm.nih.gov/pmc/articles/PMC6146358/.

"Homemade Burgers vs. Fast-food Burgers: How to Make the Healthier Choice," Kitchenware Rater, August 7, 2021, https://kitchenwarerater.com/homemade-burgers-vs-fast-food-burgers/.

Joslyn Brenton, Sarah Bowen, Sinikka Elliott, "Time to Cook Is a Luxury Many Families Don't Have," *The Conversation*, June 19, 2019, https://theconversation.com/time-to-cook-is-a-luxury-many-families-dont-have-117158.

Rachael Link, "Top 10 Healthy Cuisines from Around the World," Healthline, Nov. 12, 2021, https://www.healthline.com/health/food-nutrition/travel-healthiest-cuisines.

Roni Caryn Rabin, "Why Is Fish Good for You? Because It Replaces Meat?," *New York Times*, October 7, 2016, https://well.blogs.nytimes.com/2016/10/07/why-is-fish-good-for-you-because-it-replaces-meat/.

"Advice about Eating Fish," U.S. Food and Drug Administration, https://www.fda.gov/media/102331/download.

"Lead in Drinking Water," Centers for Disease Control and Prevention, https://www.cdc.gov/nceh/lead/prevention/sources/water.htm.

Dr. Michael Mosley, "Should I Worry about Arsenic in My Rice?," *BBC News*, February 10, 2017, https://www.bbc.com/news/health-38910848.

"Does Metabolism Matter In Weight Loss?," Harvard Health Publishing, https://www.health.harvard.edu/diet-and-weight-loss/does-metabolism-matter-in-weight-loss.

Lisa Drayer, "Do Skinny People Have Faster Metabolisms? Not Really," *CNN Health*, https://www.cnn.com/2019/03/07/health/skinny-metabolism-food-drayer/index.html.

"Weight Management: State of the Science and Opportunities for Military Programs," National Academy of Sciences, https://www.ncbi.nlm.nih.gov/books/NBK221834/.

"Do You Know These Surprising Health Facts?," Spectrum Health Care, September 17, 2019, https://spectrumhealthcare.com/resources/do-you-know-these-surprising-health-facts/.

"How Laughter Benefits Your Heart Health," Henry Ford Health System, March 5, 2019, https://www.henryford.com/blog/2019/03/how-laughter-benefits-heart-health.

"Foods Linked to Better Brainpower," Harvard Health Publishing, March 6, 2021, https://www.health.harvard.edu/healthbeat/foods-linked-to-better-brainpower.

"40 Easy Ways to Burn Extra Calories Every Day," Eat This, Not That!, October 13, 2021, https://www.eatthis.com/easy-ways-to-burn-calories/.

"Calorie Burn Rate Calculator," University of Rochester Medical Center, https://www.urmc.rochester.edu/encyclopedia/content.aspx?ContentTypeID=41&ContentID=CalorieBurnCalc&CalorieBurnCalc_Parameters=160.

"How Many Calories Does Fidgeting Burn? Fidgeting for Weight Loss," Fitness Blender, https://www.fitnessblender.com/articles/how-many-calories-does-fidgeting-burn-fidgeting-for-weight-loss.

"Well-Known Facts: Healthy Edition," Fish of Gold, June 6, 2013, https://fishofgold.net/2013/06/06/well-known-facts-healthy-edition/.

Susan Hall, "19 Easy Ways You Can Torch 200 Calories in a Blink of an Eye," *The Healthy*, April 24, 2018, https://www.thehealthy.com/weight-loss/ways-to-torch-200-calories/.

Markham Heid, "You Asked: How Many Calories Does Sex Burn?," *Time*, August 9, 2017, https://time.com/4891579/how-many-calories-does-sex-burn/.

Luke Ward, "20 Bizarre Ways to Burn Calories," The Fact Site, August 7, 2021, https://www.thefactsite.com/20-bizarre-ways-to-burn-calories/.

Claudia Hammond, "Should You Put Butter on a Burn?," BBC, August 19, 2013, https://www.bbc.com/future/article/20130820-should-you-put-butter-on-a-burn.

Rosa Escandon, "9 Home Remedies Backed by Science," Healthline, July 29, 2019, https://www.healthline.com/health/home-remedies.

An Inside Scoop on the Science Behind Chicken Soup and the Common Cold, UCLA: Explore IM, https://exploreim.ucla.edu/wellness/an-inside-scoop-on-the-science-behind-chicken-soup-and-the-common-cold/.

"Medical Communication Companies and Industry Grants," *JAMA*, December 18, 2013, https://jamanetwork.com/journals/jama/fullarticle/1790870.

Julie Beck, "Online Symptom Checkers Are Often Wrong (Phew)," *The Atlantic*, July 16, 2015, https://www.theatlantic.com/health/archive/2015/07/online-symptom-checkers-inaccurate-webmd/398654/.

"Causes of Common Headaches, Harvard Health Publishing, February 3, 2021, https://www.health.harvard.edu/staying-healthy/causes-of-headaches.

Jillian Kubala, MD, RD, "18 Remedies to Get Rid of Headaches Naturally," Healthline, February 4, 2018, https://www.healthline.com/nutrition/headache-remedies.

"Know Your Headaches," Cedars-Sinai, February 8, 2018, https://www.cedars-sinai.org/blog/know-your-headaches.html.

"The Frequency of Diagnostic Errors in Outpatient Care: Estimations from Three Large Observational Studies Involving U.S. Adult Populations," *BMJ Journals*, vol. 23, issue 9, https://qualitysafety.bmj.com/content/23/9/727.

Heidi Godman, "What to Do When You Disagree With Your Doctor," *U.S. News & World Report*, August 24, 2018, https://health.usnews.com/health-care/patient-advice/articles/2018-08-24/what-to-do-when-you-disagree-with-your-doctor.

Sandy Cohen, "The Fastest Vaccine in History," UCLA Health, December 10, 2020, https://connect.uclahealth.org/2020/12/10/the-fastest-vaccine-in-history/.

Rachel Schraer, "Cancer Drug: New Treatment Halts Tumour Growth," *BBC News*, June 23, 2020, https://www.bbc.com/news/health-53137328.

Gary Robbins, "Will Scientists Wipe Out Disease by 2030?," *San Diego Union Tribune*, November 8, 2015, https://www.sandiegouniontribune.com/sdut-ray-kurzweil-conference-2015nov08-story.html.

Tim Jewell, "Why Does My Body Ache?," Healthline, June 12, 2017, https://www.healthline.com/health/body-aches.

"Muscle Pain," Mayo Clinic, https://www.mayoclinic.org/symptoms/muscle-pain/basics/causes/sym-20050866.

"Nearly 1 in 5 Americans Haven't Seen a Doctor in over Five Years," OnlineDoctor, April 14, 2021, https://www.onlinedoctor.com/nearly-1-in-5-americans-havent-seen-a-doctor-in-over-five-years/.

Stacey Colino, "How to Make the Most of Your First Doctor's Appointment in a While," *The Washington Post*, June 18, 2021, https://www.washingtonpost.com/lifestyle/wellness/havent-seen-doctor-appointment-tips/2021/06/17/4e171f80-cf6b-11eb-8014-2f3926ca24d9_story.html.

"Chess Therapy," Theravive, https://www.theravive.com/therapedia/chess-therapy.

Marie Miguel, "4 'Strange' Types of Therapy You Probably Don't Know About," The Mighty, August 21, 2018, https://themighty.com/2018/08/strange-therapy-types/.

Dr. Martin Kalff, "On the History of ISST," ISST, International Society for Sandplay Therapy, https://www.isst-society.com/history.

Samantha Popp, "10 of the Strangest Psychotherapy Techniques," Listverse, June 11, 2015, https://listverse.com/2015/06/11/10-of-the-strangest-psychotherapy-techniques/.

Margarita Tartakovsky, "The History of Nude Psychotherapy," PsychCentral, November 18, 2011, https://psychcentral.com/blog/the-history-of-nude-psychotherapy#5.

Amanda Rife, "10 Negative Effects of Social Media That Can Harm Your Life," LifeHack, updated April 19, 2021, https://www.lifehack.org/articles/technology/you-should-aware-these-10-effects-social-media-you.html.

Amy Fleming, "Why Social Media Makes Us so Angry, and What You Can Do about It," *BBC Science Focus Magazine*, April 2, 2020, https://www.sciencefocus.com/the-human-body/why-social-media-makes-us-so-angry-and-what-you-can-do-about-it/.

Carmella de los Angeles Guiol, "I Gave Up All Social Media for One Full Year. Here's My Report from the Other Side," *Self*, https://www.self.com/story/social-media-sabbatical.

Jennifer Dene, "Squashing Overwhelm & Reaching Your Goals," Jennifer Dene Wellness, http://www.jenniferdenewellness.com/healthy-lifestyle/.

Jody Michael, MCC, BCC, "Overwhelmed by Wellness?," Jody Michael, https://www.jodymichael.com/blog/overwhelmed-by-wellness/.

Michael Precker, "Enjoy Your Nap, but Be Aware of the Pros and Cons," American Heart Association News, July 22, 2020, https://www.heart.org/en/news/2020/07/22/enjoy-your-nap-but-be-aware-of-the-pros-and-cons.

Shelby Freedman Harris, PsyD, "The Pros and Cons of Napping," *HuffPost*, August 23, 2013, https://www.huffpost.com/entry/daytime-napping_n_3757655.

Jane Porter, "Routine Disruption: How to Change Your Habits for the Better," Help Scout, https://www.helpscout.com/blog/disrupt-daily-routine/.

Kathleen Smith, PhD, LPC, "The Psychology of Dealing With Change: How to Become Resilient," PsyCom, https://www.psycom.net/dealing-with-change.

"The Unexpected Benefits of Shaking Up Your Work Routine," Medium, January 31, 2017, https://medium.com/work-life-success/https-medium-com-wrike-the-4-benefits-of-shaking-up-your-routines-fcdd5b27fa28.

Elissa Bertot, "How to Take Your Own Advice (and Why It's So Damn Hard)," Favor the Bold Communications, https://favortheboldcommunications.com/blog/take-advice.

Polly Campbell, "Should You Take Your Own Advice?," *Psychology Today*, June 18, 2019, https://www.psychologytoday.com/us/blog/imperfect-spirituality/201906/should-you-take-your-own-advice.

Dan Gordon and Justin Roberts, "This Is How Long It Takes Your Body to Fall Out of Shape When You Stop Exercising," *CNN Health*, updated May 31, 2021, https://www.cnn.com/2021/05/31/health/unfit-working-out-wellness-partner/index.html.

Alyssa Petersel, "What to Do When It Feels Like the World Is Ending," My Wellbeing, March 18, 2020, https://mywellbeing.com/ask-a-therapist/what-to-do-when-it-feels-like-the-world-is-ending.

Utpal Dholakia, PhD, "4 Reasons Why an Optimistic Outlook Is Good for Your Health," *Psychology Today*, July 31, 2016, https://www.psychologytoday.com/us/blog/the-science-behind-behavior/201607/4-reasons-why-optimistic-outlook-is-good-your-health.

Julia K. Boehm and Laura D, Kubzansky, "The Heart's Content: The Association between Positive Psychological Well-being and Cardiovascular Health," APA PsycNet, https://doi.org/10.1037/a0027448.

Nina Garcia, "Why Parenting Is Harder than Your Day Job," Sleeping Should Be Easy, September 12, 2020, https://sleepingshouldbeeasy.com/hardest-job/.

"Dad Advice: How to Unwind after Work," Life of Dad, https://www.lifeofdad.com/dad-advice-how-to-unwind-after-work/.

David Sturt and Todd Nordstrom, "Bored at Work? Science Says That's a Good Thing," *Forbes*, May 24, 2018, https://www.forbes.com/sites/davidsturt/2018/05/24/bored-at-work-science-says-thats-a-good-thing/.

Leon Ho, "What to Do When Bored at Work (and Why You Feel Bored Actually)," Lifehack, December 15, 2020, https://www.lifehack.org/572501/feeling-bored-work-here-are-causes-you-may-not-realize-and-how-you-can-cure-the-boredom.

"What to Do When You Are Feeling Incompetent at Work," Indeed, March 25, 2021, https://www.indeed.com/career-advice/career-development/feeling-incompetent-at-work.

Tomas Chamorro-Premuzic, "The Psychological Benefits and Drawbacks of Perfectionism," *Fast Company*, September 15, 2015, https://www.fastcompany.com/3050989/a-psychologist-breaks-down-the-pros-and-cons-of-perfectionism.

"STRESS . . . at Work," Centers for Disease Control and Prevention, https://www.cdc.gov/niosh/docs/99-101/default.html.

"Coping with Stress at Work," American Psychological Association, updated October 14, 2018, https://www.apa.org/topics/healthy-workplaces/work-stress.

"How to Keep Work Stress from Taking Over Your Life," Healthline, https://www.healthline.com/health/work-stress#rely-on-others.

Jack Kelly, "10 Telltale Signs That Your Boss Hates You and Wants to Push You out the Door," *Forbes*, February 8, 2019, https://www.forbes.com/sites/jackkelly/2019/02/08/10-telltale-signs-that-your-boss-hates-you-and-wants-to-push-you-out-the-door/.

Jacquelyn Smith, "Here's What to Do When You Realize Your Boss Secretly Hates You," *Insider*, January 29, 2016, https://www.businessinsider.com/what-to-do-when-you-realize-your-boss-secretly-hates-you-2016-1.

"What Percentage of Our Lives Are Spent Working?," Reference, March 24, 2020, https://www.reference.com/world-view/percentage-lives-spent-working-599e3f7fb2c88fca.

"15 Workplace Exercises to Keep You Healthy at the Office," Indeed, February 22, 2021, https://www.indeed.com/career-advice/career-development/workplace-exercise.

Gabrielle Moss, "Is Fluorescent Lighting Bad for You?," Bustle, August 14, 2015, https://www.bustle.com/articles/104264-is-fluorescent-light-bad-for-you-3-things-you-should-know-about-the-common-office-lighting.

Matt Brady, "Benefits of Natural Light in the Workplace," New Day Office, https://www.newdayoffice.com/blog/benefits-of-natural-light-in-the-workplace.

Jeanne C. Meister, "The #1 Office Perk? Natural Light," *Harvard Business Review*, September 3, 2018, https://hbr.org/2018/09/the-1-office-perk-natural-light.

"Workers Compensation Deadlines: All 50 States," Work Injury Source, https://workinjurysource.com/what-you-need-to-know/state-workers-compensation-resources/workers-compensation-deadlines-50-states/.

"Why Is It Important for All Work Injuries to be Reported?," Lawteryx, July 19, 2018, https://www.lawteryx.com/blog/workers-compensation-employment-law/reasons-report-injury-promptly.htm.

Philip Ellis, "This Guy Built a Gym Out of Wood So He Could Get 'Lumber Jacked' in Quarantine," *Men's Health*, April 9, 2020, https://www.menshealth.com/fitness/a32094780/quarantine-home-workout-wood-gym-lumber-jacked-facebook/.

Olivia Saccameno, "Fitness Gimmicks: 15 Unforgettable (& Ridiculous) Exercise Products," ActiveCities, http://activecities.com/blog/fitness-gimmicks-15-unforgettable-and-ridiculous-exercise-products/.

Jordan Shakeshaft, "The 17 Biggest Fitness Fads That Flopped," Greatist, January 30, 2012, https://greatist.com/fitness/17-biggest-fitness-fads-flopped#1.

"15 of the Worst Fitness Products Still Selling Online," Fit Dad Nation, https://www.fitdadnation.com/15-worst-fitness-products/.

Christina Stiehl, "Ridiculous Fitness Equipment That Never Should've Existed," Thrillist, September 16, 2016, https://www.thrillist.com/health/nation/ridiculous-fitness-equipment-that-should-never-have-existed.

Malia Frey, "How to Start a Workout Routine If You're Overweight," *Verywell Fit*, February 25, 2021, https://www.verywellfit.com/best-workouts-if-youre-overweight-3495993.

Jessica Timmons, "How Sedentary Obese People Can Ease into Regular Exercise," Healthline, updated December 18, 2016, https://www.healthline.com/health/fitness-exercise/exercise-for-obese-people.

Lori Smith, MSN, BSN, WHNP-BC, "How Can Physical Therapy Help?," Medical News Today, March 8, 2017, https://www.medicalnewstoday.com/articles/160645.

Gregory L. Jantz, PhD, "6 Signs That You're Addicted to Something," *Psychology Today*, November 5, 2014, https://www.psychologytoday.com/us/blog/hope-relationships/201411/6-signs-youre-addicted-something.

Mara Tyler, "Recognizing an Addiction Problem," Healthline, January 12, 2018, https://www.healthline.com/health/addiction/recognizing-addiction.

Elizabeth Hartney, BSc, MSc, MA, PhD, "How to Stop an Addiction," Verywell Mind, September 1, 2021, https://www.verywellmind.com/how-can-i-quit-my-addiction-22390.

"Addiction Counseling: When to Seek Help," Life Stance Health, March 2, 2017, https://advancedcounseling.info/addiction-counseling-seek-help/.

Terri Williams, "Don't Have Health Insurance? What's the Worst That Could Happen?," Investopedia, September 7, 2021, https://www.investopedia.com/articles/personal-finance/120815/dont-have-health-insurance-whats-worst-could-happen.asp.

Lorie Konish, "This Is the Real Reason Most Americans File for Bankruptcy," CNBC, updated February 11, 2019, https://www.cnbc.com/2019/02/11/this-is-the-real-reason-most-americans-file-for-bankruptcy.html.

"Health Coverage Options if You're Unemployed," HealthCare.gov, https://www.healthcare.gov/unemployed/coverage/.

"Depression," World Health Organization, September 13, 2021, https://www.who.int/news-room/fact-sheets/detail/depression.

Melinda Smith, MA, Lawrence Robinson, and Jeanne Segal, PhD, "Coping with Depression," HelpGuide, October 2021, https://www.helpguide.org/articles/depression/coping-with-depression.htm.

Katie Hurley, LCSW, "Coping with Depression: How to Find Help," PsyCom, updated March 18, 2019, https://www.psycom.net/depression-where-to-find-help.

Kate Sweeny and Michael D. Dooley, "The Surprising Upsides of Worry," Wiley Online Library, April 18, 2017, https://onlinelibrary.wiley.com/doi/abs/10.1111/spc3.12311.

Charlotte Hilton Anderson, "Yes, It's OK to Worry Sometimes—If You Do It Right. Here's Why," The Healthy, July 10, 2017, https://www.thehealthy.com/mental-health/worrying-ok-do-it-right/.

Agata Blaszczak-Boxe, "Don't Worry If You're a Worrier . . . It Could Be Good for You," Live Science, May 3, 2017, https://www.livescience.com/58951-why-worrying-can-be-good-for-you.html

ABOUT THE AUTHOR

David Vienna is the mastermind behind the popular parenting social media entity The Daddy Complex. His viral post "The CTFD Method" catalyzed his success, which he followed up with his debut book *Calm the F*ck Down*, a bestseller that was named the #1 Best Baby Book for New and Expecting Parents by *Women's Health* magazine. He followed that book with send-ups of pop culture, parenting, and politics: *Drinks for Mundane Tasks*, a cocktail recipe book for those with a to-do list; *Are We There Yet?*, a flowchart book for parents stumped by their kids' "bad decisions"; and *Anyone Can Be President*, an interactive guide to campaigning for and being the leader of the free world. He also wrote the independent film *More Than Stars*, the horror podcast *Barren*, and exquisitely crafted drunken emails to his friends from high school.